Hughes'
Outline
of
Modern Psychiatry

Fourth Edition

Wiley Titles of Related Interest...

BIOLOGICAL PSYCHIATRY
Second Edition

M.R. TRIMBLE

Written by a leading expert, this new edition reflects the major advances which have occurred in the field of biological psychiatry. Providing a fully updated and authoritative text on the subject, it is presented in a new easy-to-read format. An indispensable reference work, it will appeal to a wide, international audience in the fields of psychiatry, psychology and mental health

0471 96360 7   480pp   1996   Cloth
0471 95374 1   480pp   1996   Paperback

PSYCHOPHARMACOLOGY
An Introduction
Third Edition

R. SPIEGEL

Completely updated and revised, the third edition of this highly successful book incorporates many of the latest developments in the field of psychopharmacology. An introduction to modern psychopharmaceuticals, their therapeutic uses and limitations, adverse reactions and future directions for research, its emphasis is very much clinical and psychological.

0471 95729 1   312pp   1996   Cloth

MODELS FOR MENTAL DISORDER
Conceptual Models in Psychiatry
Second Edition

P. TYRER and D. STEINBERG

"This compact text outlines the different models underpinning schools of psychiatric thought highlighting advantages and differences. An excellent background introduction to the field for all health workers."

Journal of the Institute of Health Education

0471 93983 8   158pp   1993   Paparback

Hughes'
Outline
of
Modern Psychiatry

Fourth Edition

JENNIFER BARRACLOUGH
Sir Michael Sobell House
Churchill Hospital, Oxford, UK

and

DAVID GILL
Institute of Health Sciences
Anglia & Oxford Regional Health Authority, Oxford, UK

JOHN WILEY & SONS
Chichester · New York · Brisbane · Toronto · Singapore

Copyright © 1996 by John Wiley & Sons Ltd,
Baffins Lane, Chichester,
West Sussex PO19 1UD, England

National   01243 779777
International   (+44) 1243 779777

Other Wiley Editorial Offices

John Wiley & Sons, Inc., 605 Third Avenue,
New York, NY 10158-0012, USA

Jacaranda Wiley Ltd, 33 Park Road, Milton,
Queensland 4064, Australia

John Wiley & Sons (Canada) Ltd, 22 Worcester Road,
Rexdale, Ontario M9W 1L1, Canada

John Wiley & Sons (Asia) Pte Ltd, 2 Clementi Loop #02-01
Jin Xing Distripark, Singapore 0512

Library of Congress Cataloging-in-Publication Data

Barraclough, Jennifer.
    Hughes' outline of modern psychiatry / Jennifer Barraclough and
David Gill. — 4th ed.
        p.   cm.
    Rev. ed. of: An outline of modern psychiatry / Jennifer Hughes. 3rd
ed. c1991.
    Includes bibliographical references and index.
    ISBN 0-471-96358-5 (paper : alk. paper)
    1. Psychiatry—Handbooks, manuals, etc.   I. Gill, David, Dr.
II. Barraclough, Jennifer Outline of modern psychiatry.
III. Title.
    [DNLM: 1. Mental Disorders—handbooks.   WM 34 B268h 1996]
RC456.H84   1996
616.89—dc20
DNLM/DLC
for Library of Congress   95–50016
                                                           CIP
British Library Cataloguing in Publication Data

A catalogue record for this book is available from the British Library

ISBN 0-471-96358-5

Typeset in 11/13 pt Palatino from the authors' disks by Saxon Graphics Ltd, Derby
Printed and bound in Great Britain by Biddles Ltd, Guildford and Kings Lynn
This book is printed on acid-free paper responsibly manufactured from sustainable forestation,
for which at least two trees are planted for each one used for paper production.

Contents

PART III: TREATMENT

Preface

I wrote the first edition of *An Outline of Modern Psychiatry* in the late 1970s, when preparing to take my MRCPsych examination. The book was intended to summarise current knowledge of the subject in a concise way, concentrating on fact rather than theory, using a format suitable for quick reference or revision. Originally intended for medical students and trainee psychiatrists as an adjunct to longer texts, it proved to appeal to a wider audience including GPs, MRCP candidates, nurses, clinical psychologists and social workers, also some general readers.

For this fourth edition I have been pleased to enlist the help of Dr David Gill as co-author to share the task of up-dating the book without adding too much to its length. We have had to be selective in choosing new material from the large volume of recently published research, the changes in classification and terminology, and the innovations in methods of NHS service delivery. Rather than rearrange the order of topics to correspond with ICD-10, we have retained more or less the same chapter headings which were used in previous editions of the book.

For reasons of confidentiality, the clinical examples are made up of composite case histories and do not refer to real individual patients.

JENNIFER BARRACLOUGH (*formerly Hughes*) 1995

Acknowledgements

We are most grateful to Cecilia Batten, Don Batten, Steve Brown, Dan Harwood and Dermot Rowe for reviewing some of the chapters; to Maureen Heath and Meg Roberts for help with the manuscript and references; and to Brian Barraclough for numerous constructive suggestions on the project as a whole.

I
The Nature and Assessment of Psychiatric Disorder

1
Classification

Psychiatry is the branch of medicine which deals with mental, emotional and behavioural disorders. In psychiatry, as in other branches of medicine, classification of disease is useful for:

- *Informing clinical practice*: by placing a given patient's disorder into a recognised diagnostic category, the clinician is able to make an appropriate choice of treatment, and judge the probable future outcome. Using a classification system in this way does not, of course, remove the need to consider and respect those features which are unique to each individual case.
- *Communication between professionals*: a universally understood classification system permits efficient communication, whether in everyday clinical practice when colleagues are discussing a case, or in the national and international literature.
- *A basis for research*: research workers require a classification system in order to investigate the causes, clinical features, natural history and response to treatment of the various psychiatric disorders.
- *Service planning*: the type of treatment services required in a given area will depend on the frequency of different disorders within the local population.

THE BASIS OF CLASSIFICATION

The most rigorous type of classification is one based on cause, for example a single gene defect (Huntington's disease) or an infection (neurosyphilis).

However, for most psychiatric disorders this is inapplicable, and so official psychiatric classification systems largely consist of descriptive accounts of clinical syndromes each with their characteristic symptoms, signs and natural history.

RELIABILITY AND VALIDITY

Reliability: a diagnosis may be said to be reliable if the same observer reaches the same diagnosis in a repeat of the same clinical situation (test-retest reliability), or if two observers reach the same diagnosis in the same clinical situation (inter-rater reliability).

Studies in clinical practice have often showed low reliability for psychiatric diagnosis because psychiatrists differ in the way they interview patients and interpret the information elicited. Diagnostic practices also vary between different parts of the world. Reliability is better for individual symptoms and signs.

Reliability can be improved by using standardised interviews and questionnaires (Ch 3), and operational criteria like those in ICD-10 and DSM-IV (see below). This is necessary for research purposes, but too time-consuming to be a usual part of daily clinical practice.

Validity of a diagnosis is more difficult to ascertain. If a classification is to be valid ("based on truth or correct reasoning"), the categories it contains should describe disorders which really are separate from one another. Ways of testing the validity of diagnostic groupings include:

- Examining the consistency of symptom patterns. Statistical techniques such as "cluster analysis" and "discriminant function analysis" facilitate this process.
- Demonstration of consistent genetic and biological correlates.
- Demonstration of a consistent natural history and long-term outcome.
- Demonstration of a consistent treatment response.

LIMITATIONS AND PROBLEMS OF CLASSIFICATION

Although a great deal of work has been devoted to making the official international classification systems both reliable and valid, it must be acknowledged that they are still imperfect. The descriptive categories are continually being revised, for example "panic disorder" and "post-traumatic stress disorder" were only recently listed as diagnoses, although the clinical phenomena have been recognised for many years.

The boundaries between some of the clinical syndromes are not absolute, as illustrated by the need for terms like "schizo-affective disorder" to describe an illness with mixed features of two supposedly discrete categories, "schizophrenia" and "affective disorder". Some patients' symptoms do not fit well with any recognised category and there is a danger these may be forced into a "dustbin" category such as "depression, not otherwise specified". In the USA, this may make the difference between receiving care or not, as insurers may restrict cover to certain "hard" diagnostic categories.

Insensitive use of classification can lead to "labelling" of patients. Classification systems are best used in a flexible and critical way, and clinical effort is often better directed towards relieving the patient's symptoms than excessive debate about the niceties of diagnosis. Some mental health professionals prefer "problem-based" rather than "disease-based" care.

COMMON TERMS IN PSYCHIATRIC CLASSIFICATION

Organic and Functional

Psychiatric conditions are sometimes divided into *organic brain disorders*, and *functional mental illnesses*.

Organic conditions are caused by identifiable physical pathology which affects the brain, directly or indirectly, and include for example *learning disabilities* (formerly mental handicap) and the *dementias*.

Functional conditions have usually been attributed to some kind of psychological stress, although in many cases it would be more honest to say that their cause is not known.

As knowledge advances, some "functional" conditions are likely to be reclassified as "organic" (as currently may be happening for schizophrenia), and for this reason the term "organic" is not used in DSM-IV.

Psychosis and Neurosis

These terms have largely been removed from the international classifications but are still used in clinical practice.

Psychoses (for example schizophrenia, bipolar affective disorder):

- Severe illnesses.
- Symptoms outside normal experience, such as delusions and hallucinations.
- Loss of insight; subjective experience mistaken for external reality.

Neuroses (for example anxiety disorders, most cases of depression):

- More common.
- Often less severe.
- Symptoms may be understandable as an exaggeration of the normal response to stress.

Psychiatrists also deal with conditions involving abnormalities of psychological development or behaviour, for example *personality disorders, alcohol and drug misuse, sexual dysfunction* and *eating disorders*.

The descriptive study of abnormalities of mental functions such as mood, perception, thought, volition, memory or cognition is called *psychopathology*. Definitions of some of the terms commonly used in psychopathology are given in the Glossary.

CLASSIFICATION SYSTEMS

These include *categorical, dimensional* and *multiaxial* types.

Categorical: each case is allocated to one of several mutually exclusive groups. This simple method is the most suitable one for clinical settings. Categorical systems are usually used in a hierarchical way, so that each case can only receive one main diagnosis. Organic psychoses traditionally take precedence over functional psychoses, and functional psychoses over neuroses. This can lead to oversimplification of complex cases, and does not take account of "co-morbidity" in which two psychiatric diagnoses (for example, anxiety state and alcohol misuse) or a physical and a psychiatric diagnosis (for example, diabetes and depression) co-exist.

Dimensional: cases are rated on a continuous scale, or several separate continuous scales, for the characteristic(s) under study, for example depressed mood.

Multiaxial: each case is rated on several separate categorical systems each measuring a different aspect (for example psychiatric illness, personality, intelligence).

The two main classification systems in international use, ICD and DSM, will now be summarised. Both systems have recently been revised.

ICD-10

(World Health Organization 1992)

The tenth edition of the International Classification of Disease, prepared by the World Health Organization, includes a Classification of Mental and Behavioural Disorders (ICD-10). This is the official classification used in Britain. It is a descriptive classification, with main headings as follows:

F00–F09 Organic, including symptomatic, mental disorders
F10–F19 Mental and behavioural disorders due to psychoactive substance use
F20–F29 Schizophrenia, schizotypal and delusional disorders
F30–F39 Mood (affective) disorders
F40–F48 Neurotic, stress-related and somatoform disorders
F50–F59 Behavioural syndromes associated with physiological disturbances and physical factors
F60–F69 Disorders of adult personality and behaviour
F70–F79 Mental retardation
F80–F89 Disorders of psychological development
F90–F98 Behavioural and emotional disorders with onset usually occurring in childhood or adolescence
F99 Unspecified mental disorder

Each of the main categories listed above has a number of subdivisions. Diagnostic guidelines for each condition are given in the manual.

Some conditions relevant to psychiatry, for example suicide and self-inflicted injury or poisoning, are classified in other sections of the ICD.

DSM-IV

(American Psychiatric Association 1994)

The Diagnostic and Statistical Manual of Mental Disorders, Fourth Edition (DSM-IV) is the official classification system of the American Psychiatric Association, and has been influential in Britain. DSM-IV is a multiaxial system with five axes:

Axis I: Clinical syndromes
Axis II: Developmental disorders and personality disorders
Axis III: Physical disorders and conditions
Axis IV: Severity of psychosocial stressors
Axis V: Global assessment of functioning

The strength of this approach lies in its requiring any clinical syndrome to be considered against the background of the permanent features, such as personality characteristics and intellectual level, of the person concerned. Each syndrome is defined by a set of practical criteria.

The chapter headings in this book do not follow either ICD-10 or DSM-IV exactly, because the arrangement of topics has been designed to accord with British clinical practice rather than official classification systems.

FURTHER READING

Books

American Psychiatric Association (1994) *Diagnostic and Statistical Manual of Mental Disorders* (4th edn) (DSM-IV). American Psychiatric Association: Washington, DC

World Health Organization (1992) *The ICD-10 Classification of Mental and Behavioural Disorders*. World Health Organization: Geneva

Review Articles

Kendell RE (1989) Clinical validity. *Psychological Medicine* **19**: 45–55

2
Causes And Prevention

Except for a few conditions known to result directly from specific organic pathology, the cause of most psychiatric disorders appears to be multifactorial, involving the interplay of constitutional and environmental factors. These factors include genetic predisposition, personality characteristics, physical disorders, social circumstances and life experiences. Workers from different academic disciplines may favour one particular cause, making it possible to explain the same disorder using a variety of "models": medical, social, psychodynamic, cognitive or behavioural.

Distinguishing "predisposing", "precipitating" and "perpetuating" factors may be useful in individual cases. However, sometimes no cause can be found.

This chapter outlines some general principles and research techniques. More detail regarding causation of individual disorders will be given in later chapters.

GENETICS

Most psychiatric disorders run in families. This observation could be explained by genetic factors and/or by the influence of family environment. Two long-established clinical research techniques have been used to distinguish these:

- *Twin studies*:
    - comparing monozygotic with dizygotic twins

   − comparing monozygotic twins brought up together with those brought up apart.
- *Adoption studies*: examining rates of psychiatric disorder in children whose biological parents were affected but who were brought up by healthy adoptive parents, or vice versa.

Twin and adoption studies, many of which have been carried out in Scandinavia where comprehensive national records of individuals and their health are maintained, confirm a genetic predisposition for the majority of psychiatric conditions.

The "New Genetics"

Using modern techniques of molecular biology, research to identify the genes which cause, or predispose to, conditions such as Huntington's disease, schizophrenia, affective disorders and Alzheimer's disease is now in progress. These techniques are most relevant to single-gene disorders. They include the "positional cloning" and "candidate gene" approaches, carried out on blood samples. Most accurate results are obtained from large families containing several affected members. Careful clinical documentation of these families is essential.

   The localisation of defective genes, and identification of their DNA sequences and biochemical products, will have various clinical applications:

- *Diagnosis of affected or at-risk individuals*, perhaps at a pre-symptomatic stage.
- *Identification of the carrier state* for recessive conditions.
- *Genetic counselling and prenatal diagnosis* (Ch 19).
- *Treatment possibilities*, mainly theoretical at present, including:
   − development of specific drugs
   − gene replacement.

The new techniques may, in future, bring marked clinical benefit but they also raise ethical problems. There is a danger of patients' hopes being falsely raised, particularly by media features about "Discovery of the Gene for . . .", and doctors are already seeing possible negative effects.

Case Example

A man consulted his GP in distress, having just found out that his divorced ex-wife had Huntington's disease. He knew this disease was inherited, and that a test had recently become available to diagnose it in the pre-symptomatic stage. What, if anything, should he tell their 23-year-old daughter who lived with him, and who knew nothing of her mother's illness? The GP referred the man to a genetic counsellor. After prolonged discussion, in which it was explained that a test was available but preventive or symptomatic treatment was not, he decided against telling his daughter. He felt that the possibility of her finding out, through testing, that she was to develop such a disease in later life might blight her young adulthood. However, he felt that he would wish to review this decision should she later consider starting a family. He is left with the strain of carrying a secret.

NEUROCHEMISTRY

Disturbance of brain biochemistry, especially involving monoamine transmitters, appears to be present in most psychiatric disorders; though it cannot be assumed that a chemical abnormality is the cause of the disorder rather than its result. Direct studies on the brains of living patients are limited for both practical and ethical reasons. Indirect techniques of investigation include:

- *Postmortem brain studies*: these require brains to be harvested and frozen within a few hours of death. Findings may be influenced by recent medication, and the condition which caused the death, as well as by the psychiatric disorder of interest.
- *Analysis of cerebrospinal fluid (CSF), blood or urine* for precursors or metabolites of neurotransmitters. The findings are affected by many factors such as diet and exercise, and may not give an accurate reflection of concentrations in the brain itself.
- *Pharmacological studies*: inferences about the biochemical defect present in a particular disorder may be made from studies, performed on patients or on animals, of the properties of drugs which are effective in treating that disorder.

NEURORADIOLOGY

Modern brain imaging techniques (Ch 3) show abnormalities of structure and function associated with major psychiatric illness, for example ventricular enlargement in chronic schizophrenia, and altered patterns of glucose uptake in the manic and depressed phases of bipolar affective disorder.

EPIDEMIOLOGY

Epidemiological studies investigate the frequency of psychiatric disorders, their relationship to social factors, and their natural history. They are carried out on whole populations rather than individual patients.

Sources of information include:

- *Population surveys* in which every member of a defined population, or a random sample of it, is studied by interview or questionnaire.
- *GP consultation* records.
- *Case registers*, which exist in some health districts to provide information on all contacts with psychiatric services.
- *Hospital statistics.*

Frequency may be expressed as *point prevalence* (rate of disorder at one point in time) or *period prevalence* (cumulative rate through a defined period) within a population; *incidence* (rate of new cases) within a population; or *lifetime expectation* for an individual developing the condition concerned.

The results of different surveys vary greatly. Community interview surveys find the highest rates, invariably detecting many psychiatric "cases" which are not known to GPs, let alone to specialist services. GP and hospital statistics may be inaccurate because they reflect different definitions of a psychiatric "case", or variations in local treatment policies.

Most community surveys report that 10–20% of the population meet diagnostic criteria for psychiatric disorder at any one time, and that a person's lifetime risk of disorder may be as high as 50%.

Several sociodemographic variables have an association with psychiatric morbidity but the direction of cause and effect is not always clearcut, for example:

- *Sex*: women have higher rates of psychiatric disorder than men. Possible explanations include:
  - women use health services of all kinds more frequently than men. They may be more willing to acknowledge emotional complaints and seek medical treatment, whereas men tend to express their distress through other means such as antisocial behaviour or alcohol misuse
  - doctors are more likely to diagnose women's symptoms as psychiatric
  - women suffer more psychosocial stress than men because of their role in society
  - biological differences, such as genetic constitution and sex hormone profile.
- *Marital status*: for men, rates of psychiatric disorder are lower among the married than for the single, divorced or widowed. Possible explanations include:
  - married life is beneficial for men's mental health
  - men with psychiatric disorder tend to remain single
  - psychiatric disorder results in marital breakdown
  - widowhood and divorce are stressful life events which may lead to psychiatric disorder.

For women, the pattern is different. Young working-class housewives with several small children have high rates of depression and neurosis, whereas single women in paid employment have low rates.

- *Residential area*: urban areas, especially poor inner-city districts, have higher rates of psychiatric morbidity than rural areas. Possible explanations include:
  - the lack of stable social networks in inner-city areas contributes to psychiatric disorder
  - stresses of city life such as overcrowding, high crime rates and noise contribute to psychiatric disorder
  - psychiatric disorder causes people to lose their jobs and social supports and forces them to move into city slums
  - a rural environment promotes good mental health.
- *Unemployment* is associated with psychiatric disorder. Possible explanations include:
  - the socioeconomic adversity and loss of self-esteem of the unemployed contributes to psychiatric disorder
  - workers with psychiatric disorder are liable to lose their jobs.

- *Social class*: manual workers show higher psychiatric morbidity than the professional/managerial classes. Possible explanations include:
  - genetic factors
  - a stressful and unhealthy environment
  - "drift down the social scale" caused by mental illness.
- *Nationality*, and issues of *"transcultural psychiatry"*: diagnostic statistics vary around the world. Organic brain syndromes, and somatic presentations of "functional" conditions, are more common in developing societies. Suicide rates vary greatly between countries. Some of these observed differences are genuine, due to variation in biological and social factors. Others are artefactual, depending on what kinds of behaviour are considered abnormal in the culture concerned, and disappear when uniform diagnostic criteria are applied. For example, until the 1970s the diagnosis of schizophrenia was made much more frequently in the USA than the UK, but since introduction of more rigorous diagnostic criteria it appears that schizophrenia, and other major psychotic disorders, occur about equally frequently in both places, and also in most other parts of the world.

Immigrants show high psychiatric morbidity, being especially prone to develop schizophrenia and paranoid states; refugees, who have been forced to emigrate rather than doing so by choice, are most at risk. Possible explanations include:
  - pre-existing psychiatric disorder causes people to emigrate
  - stressful circumstances in the country of origin precipitate both emigration and psychiatric illness
  - "culture shock" in the new country, including strange language and customs, and discrimination against immigrants
  - overdiagnosis, due to mental health professionals' unfamiliarity with the culture of immigrant groups, and language difficulties.

INDIVIDUAL LIFE EXPERIENCE

Adverse experiences in childhood, for example losing one's mother or being sexually abused, would be expected to increase risk of psychiatric disorder in adult life and most research studies tend to confirm this long-term association. There is also evidence for a short-term effect whereby psychosocial stress in adult life can precipitate psychiatric illness in predisposed people. This effect applies both for individual *life events* of a common kind, such as family bereavement or divorce, and for extraordinary disasters (see Ch 6 on post-traumatic stress disorder). Chronic *social stresses*, such as marital difficulties or bad housing, can also contribute. In contrast, supportive *social networks*, and close confiding relationships with others, provide some protection against psychiatric disorder following adverse life events.

Life event experience may be measured by:

- *Official records* in the case of certain major events like widowhood or divorce.
- *Questionnaires*, which are relatively easy to score but involve oversimplification.
- *Standardised interviews*, such as the Life Events and Difficulties Schedule (LEDS) developed by Brown and Harris.

The effects of life experiences can only be satisfactorily investigated by prospective follow-up of people subjected to adversity, but such studies take many years to complete and are expensive. Many published studies have therefore used retrospective methods, and their interpretation is subject to error for reasons including:

- *Mistaking the direction of causality*: an event apparently precipitating an illness (for example losing a job) may really be the result of changes in the patient's behaviour during the prodromal phase of that illness.
- *Effort after meaning*: some patients unwittingly exaggerate their experience of life event stress in order to explain the illness. For example, a woman who has given birth to a genetically handicapped baby is more likely than a control to report adverse events during pregnancy.
- *Inaccurate recollection of timing* of life events in relation to illness onset.

PREVENTION OF PSYCHIATRIC DISORDER

Primary prevention is prevention of disease from developing in the first place. The following list of measures might be important for psychiatry, though hard evidence of effectiveness is not available for all of them.

- *Medical and public health measures* to avert damage to the brain:
  - genetic counselling and prenatal diagnosis (Ch 19)
  - improved care during pregnancy and childbirth
  - improved infant welfare services including immunisation
  - control of infections, such as meningitis and HIV disease
  - avoidance of nutritional deficiencies
  - reduction of alcohol and drug misuse
  - reduction of pollution such as atmospheric lead
  - prevention of accidents, and hence of head injury, for example by seat-belts and crash-helmets
  - provision of adequate housing.
- *Psychological approaches*:
  - counselling for the bereaved, divorced, and other groups known to have a high risk of illness
  - crisis intervention for victims of major trauma
  - social work with disturbed families with particular emphasis on counterbalancing adverse effects on children.

Secondary prevention is reduction of severity of disease, and prevention of relapse, by means of early detection and treatment. Early detection can be improved by the education of health professionals and the general public about psychiatric illness (as for example in the Royal College of Psychiatrists' current "Defeat Depression" campaign), and by the use of screening questionnaires (Ch 3) in medical settings. Prevention of relapse may be achieved by drug therapy, psychotherapy and/or social support for patients who have recovered from an episode of mental illness.

Tertiary prevention is reduction of the handicaps which may result from established disease, for example rehabilitation programmes to prevent institutionalisation, and community services to reduce the burden on families.

Many of the measures noted under primary prevention are outside the sphere of influence of psychiatrists. Concentrating on secondary and tertiary prevention is more practical and has the additional benefit of focusing services on those most in need.

FURTHER READING

Books

Leff JP (1989) *Psychiatry Around the Globe*: *A Transcultural View*. Royal College of Psychiatrists (Gaskell Books): London

McGuffin P, Owen MJ, O'Donovan MC, Thapar A, Gottesman II (1994) *Seminars in Psychiatric Genetics.* Gaskell: London

Paykel ES, Jenkins R (eds) (1994) *Prevention in Psychiatry.* Gaskell: London

Tyer P, Steinberg D (1993) *Models for Mental Disorder: Conceptual Models in Psychiatry* (2nd edn). Wiley: Chichester

Williams P, Wilkinson G, Rawnsley K (1988) *The Scope of Epidemiological Psychiatry.* Routledge: London

Review Articles

Baron M, Endicott J, Ott J (1990) Genetic linkage in mental illness. Limitations and prospects. *British Journal of Psychiatry* **157**: 645–647

Feldman E (1995) The new genetics in psychiatry. *Advances in Psychiatric Treatment* **1**: 109–116

3
History-taking, Examination and Investigation

Reaching a diagnosis in a psychiatric patient relies on an accurate case history, often including information from relatives or other sources, and mental state examination. Laboratory investigations are helpful in a minority of cases only.

THE PSYCHIATRIC INTERVIEW

This is designed to obtain detailed information about past life, physical health, personality, relationships and social circumstances, as well as past and present psychiatric symptoms. Such background information can help towards making the diagnosis, choosing appropriate treatment, deciding whether the case should be managed on an inpatient or outpatient basis, and setting realistic goals.

In addition, experience of psychiatry affords a good opportunity to improve the practitioner's own interviewing and communication skills; the training will often include the use of video recordings.

The first interview plays an important part in establishing the relationship between patient and psychiatrist, and therefore has a therapeutic function as well as an information-gathering one. The interviewer must reach the best compromise between listening to the patient's own concerns, and asking the requisite factual questions. Some patients, for example those who are very anxious, need some time to talk freely before they can cooperate with more structured inquiry. Open-ended questions ("How have you been sleeping lately?") are preferable to leading ones ("Have you been waking up early?").

The interview should start with the presenting complaint, though the order of the other components may vary. It is important to include all the sections but a common-sense approach is called for; there is little use exploring the fine details of symptomatology but failing to find out that the patient has just been evicted from his or her accommodation or is about to appear in court. It is usual to take notes during the interview since there is too much material to recall accurately afterwards.

Assessment may take place in an outpatient clinic, in general practice, the patient's home, a general hospital or another site such as a police station. Privacy is important, and most psychiatrists prefer to see the patient alone, although occasional exceptions are necessary, for example if the patient is potentially violent or likely to make allegations against the practitioner. Examination candidates are allowed one hour to assess a new case. Complex cases ideally need longer than this, whereas emergencies may have to be assessed more quickly. If the patient is too ill or uncooperative to give a history, concentrate on the Mental State Examination.

The assessment is incomplete until another informant, usually a relative or friend, has been interviewed; this is especially true for cases of psychotic illness or organic brain disease. The patient's prior consent is required except in special circumstances. Where language barriers exist, the help of an interpreter may be required.

A letter summarising the assessment interview is normally sent to the patient's general practitioner, copies being filed in the casenotes and sometimes sent to other professional agencies. One side of A4 paper in single-space type is a suitable length. Issues of confidentiality may cause problems, so it is important to ensure the patient knows about the letter, who will receive a copy, and whether any sensitive personal material is to be included. Remember that patients now have the right to read their medical notes.

History

Begin by explaining who you are, and outlining the purpose, format and length of interview. For example, shake hands, invite the patient to sit down, and say "My name is Paula Johnson, I am a psychiatrist working with your consultant, Dr Jones. We have about an hour to get an idea of your problems and what help we could offer." The material may then be presented as follows:

- *Introduction*: name, age, marital status, occupation, where seen and how referred. For inpatients, legal status: whether informal or on a "section" of the Mental Health Act 1983 (if so, which one).
- *Complaints*: in patient's own words.
- *History of present illness*:
  - symptoms, including changes in sleep, appetite, mood, energy and concentration
  - duration
  - possible precipitating factors
  - effect of illness on lifestyle, relationships, working ability
  - treatment so far.

Note: if the disorder is a recurrent one, concentrate on the latest episode here, leaving the rest for "past psychiatric history".

- *Past psychiatric history*: previous episodes of illness with dates, precipitating factors, symptoms, diagnosis, treatment.
- *Medical history*: past illnesses, present physical symptoms, medication.
- *Family history*:
  - parents' and siblings' ages, occupation, health, and relationship with patient. If dead, record cause of death, age at death, and patient's age at the time
  - family history of psychiatric illness (the term "nervous breakdown" may be useful), suicide, alcoholism.

Note: this section is concerned with family of origin. Spouse and children come later.

- *Childhood*:
  - complications during pregnancy or birth, serious illness in infancy, or delays in development
  - home environment: place of birth, subsequent changes of residence, emotional atmosphere and practical circumstances at home, outstanding events
  - school: academic achievements, ability to mix with other children, attitude to teachers.
- *Work*: training and qualifications, jobs held, reasons for change,

extent of satisfaction with work and ability to cope, relations with workmates and employers.

- *Sex and marriage*:
  - sexual practice: hetero- and homosexual experience, extent of satisfaction, sexual difficulties, any past history of sexual abuse
  - marital: duration of marriage/cohabitation, partner's age, occupation, health, and relationship with patient. For any previous marriages or long-term relationships, record duration and reasons for ending
  - children: names, ages, health, relationships with patient
  - for women: live births, stillbirths, miscarriages, abortions, contraceptive practice, menstrual pattern.

Note: use judgement about the extent of questioning on sexual topics. For some patients, detailed questioning is not relevant and may cause offence.

- *Premorbid personality*:
  - social relations: ability to make friends and relate to those in authority
  - mood: cheerful or despondent, anxious or placid, tendency to mood swings, way of expressing anger, response to stress
  - character: confident or diffident, independent or reliant on others, conscientious or casual, impulsive or cautious
  - level of energy and activity
  - attitude to religion, politics, membership of societies, hobbies
  - alcohol, caffeine, smoking, use of recreational drugs
  - criminal behaviour.

In some patients, the presenting disturbance is an exaggeration of longstanding personality problems. In others, recent alteration of mood and behaviour suggest psychiatric illness.

Note: many patients cannot describe their previous personality accurately and an account from another informant is often useful.

- *Present circumstances*: type of accommodation, people in household, financial or practical problems.

Note: parts of the illness not concerned with the present illness are called the "personal history".

MENTAL STATE EXAMINATION

As an objective assessment of the patient's present condition, made by a trained observer, this is especially important if there is any doubt as to the completeness or reliability of the history.

- *Introduction*: mentioning quality of rapport and interview, for example "This was a difficult interview because the patient was unforthcoming, and we did not establish a warm rapport."
- *Appearance and general behaviour*: use factual descriptions rather than judgemental comments.
    - striking physical features (such as extremes of height or weight, deformities)
    - type of dress
    - standard of self-care
    - degree of activity
    - abnormalities of movement or gait
    - whether cooperative.
- *Talk*:
    - amount
    - speed
    - spontaneous, or only in answer to questions
    - unusual features such as puns, rhymes, odd changes of topic or abrupt pauses.

Write down a sample of talk if the form is abnormal.

- *Mood*: include both patient's own description and interviewer's observations.
    - mood states include depression, euphoria, anxiety, perplexity, fear, suspicion
    - lability of mood: mood fluctuates during interview
    - mood incongruence: inappropriate to circumstances or thought content.
- *Thought*:
    - content: subjects which preoccupy the patient
    - disorders of possession (for example thought broadcasting)
    - formal thought disorder (disordered connection between thoughts).
- *Abnormal beliefs and experiences*:
    - delusions (false beliefs)
    - perceptual disorders, including depersonalisation/derealisation, hallucinations (false perceptions), illusions.

Note: the above terms are defined in the Glossary. Auditory hallucinations, which are common in psychiatric inpatients, can be covered by direct inquiry about hearing voices. Delusions, by definition, cannot be asked about directly but may be elicited by tactful exploration of any odd statements already made, or asking the patient's opinion about the cause of the presenting problems.

- *Obsessive and compulsive phenomena* (Ch 6)
- *Cognitive function*:
  - *memory*: long-term memory can be assessed from the history. Tests of short-term memory include repeating a name and address both immediately and after five minutes, and the digit span test (most people can remember a 5-digit number). Questions about general information should be fitted to the patient's age and education. Naming the monarch, the Prime Minister and the president of the USA are too easy for most. Other tests might include naming six large towns, or recalling items of current affairs
  - *orientation*: in time (day, date, time of day), place, and person (identifying the interviewer, or ward staff)
  - *attention and concentration*: tests include listing the months of the year in reverse order, and subtracting "serial sevens" from 100 (93, 86, 79, 72 etc.)
  - *intelligence*, as estimated by the interviewer.

Note: do not be tempted to miss out cognitive testing, which may reveal unsuspected defects pointing to organic cerebral dysfunction. Cognitive testing should always be done in examinations.

- *Insight*: avoid meaningless statements such as "partial insight present", but consider practical questions such as: does the patient believe an illness is present, or attribute all the symptoms to an external cause (such as poisoning by rays)? Will the patient accept treatment?

Note: not all patients referred to psychiatrists are mentally ill! Apparent paranoid delusions, for example, may reflect real persecution.

PHYSICAL EXAMINATION

All inpatients should have a physical examination, including a thorough neurological one. For outpatients, responsibility for physical examination is generally accepted as remaining with the referrer, however it is good practice to check for physical signs relevant to the case; for example to look for signs of thyrotoxicosis in a patient with symptoms of anxiety, for injection marks in a patient with suspected intravenous drug use, or for extrapyramidal signs in a patient on antipsychotic drugs. Examination candidates should always check for selected physical signs such as these.

Appraisal

The appraisal of a new case includes:

- The *positive features* of history and examination.
- Any *relevant negative features*, for example absence of a family history.
- *Differential diagnoses*, starting with the most likely possibility, and giving evidence for and against each one. A definite diagnosis cannot always be made from the first interview, so listing two or three possibilities is quite acceptable.
- *Aetiology*, considering predisposing, precipitating and perpetuating factors, and the question of why the disorder has developed at this stage in the patient's life.
- Plan of *investigation*, for example interview with informant, selected laboratory tests.
- Plan of *management*.
- Comments on *prognosis*.

Case Example 1

A single man aged 26, who has been unemployed since he dropped out of art college five years ago, and who lives with his mother. He was admitted to the psychiatric hospital under Section 2 of the Mental Health Act 1983, after trying to jump from an underground platform but being pulled back by another passenger. He did this because he kept hearing two voices talking to each other, saying "foul things" about him. He says his problems began six months ago when he saw the girl he wanted to marry (though he had never spoken to her) going into a pub with another man. Since then he has felt low in mood, lost interest in everything and stayed in his room most of the day, had both early and late insomnia and not wanted to eat because the food tasted different. He admits to smoking cannabis several times a week for several years.

On examination he was a thin man, casually dressed. He seemed suspicious, and several times he suddenly stopped talking in mid-sentence and looked round as if he had heard something behind him. He described depressive symptoms and third-person auditory hallucinations as above.

Differential diagnosis includes schizophrenia; depressive illness; and drug-induced psychosis.

Predisposing factors include genetic loading for psychiatric disorder, because the patient's father has had several admissions to a mental hospital and now has injections from a community nurse.

Further investigations should include a physical examination; urine screen for drugs; an interview with the patient's mother; and perusal of his father's notes. Initial management will include close observation in the ward setting, bearing in mind a possible continuing suicide risk.

Case Example 2

A 37-year-old married man who was referred to psychiatric outpatients from the gastroenterology clinic where he has been attending for two years with a diagnosis of irritable bowel syndrome. Recent physical investigations have not shown any new pathology. His symptoms of abdominal pain and diarrhoea have been worse over the past six months, since he was made redundant from work. During this time he has also developed low mood, poor appetite with weight loss, loss of libido, and insomnia with early waking. On mental state examination he appeared anxious and depressed; borborygmi were audible during the interview, and the patient had to leave at one point to visit the lavatory.

The most likely diagnosis is a depressive illness, with associated anxiety symptoms, and exacerbation of his functional bowel disorder. The diagnosis of anxiety disorder alone could not explain his biological symptoms. Another possibility is organic bowel disease but this seems unlikely in view of his recent normal investigations. He appears predisposed to psychological disorder by an anxious personality, and this present episode appeared precipitated by his redundancy and perpetuated by his continuing unemployment.

An interview with his wife confirmed the likely diagnosis of depression, and suggested that the patient had been particularly affected by his loss of role as breadwinner for the family, because his wife had recently been promoted in her own work.

Further physical investigation seems unnecessary, and might even prove unhelpful by adding to the patient's worries about his physical health. Antidepressant medication would be the quickest way to help this man, and amitryptiline would be suitable with its additional sedative, anxiolytic and hypnotic properties. He could also be offered training in psychological techniques of anxiety management.

STRUCTURED INTERVIEWS AND QUESTIONNAIRES

These instruments are used mainly in research work. Their purpose is collection of data in a reliable standard form, minimising the bias which can arise from variation in individual interview technique. They can be administered by trained personnel other than psychiatrists.

Well-known examples of structured interviews are the *Present State Examination* (PSE) and its later development the *Schedules for Clinical Assessment in Neuropsychiatry* (SCAN) which is analysed by computer (CATEGO programme) to produce a diagnosis; the *Standardised Psychiatric Interview* (SPI) or *Clinical Interview Schedule* (CIS) developed for use in general practice and concerned largely with neurotic symptoms; and the *Structured Clinical Interview for DSM-IV* (SCID).

A widely-used questionnaire is the *General Health Questionnaire* (GHQ), a self-rating instrument used to detect probable cases of psychiatric disorder in general practice settings or community surveys. Many other questionnaires, both self-rating and observer-rating, exist for specific parameters such as depression, anxiety or cognitive impairment.

Computer programmes for direct self-assessment of patients have been used in research projects and found to be valid, acceptable and cost-effective for certain psychiatric conditions, but seem unlikely to replace clinical interviews in everyday practice.

PSYCHOLOGICAL AND SOCIAL INVESTIGATIONS

Interview with Informant

A separate interview with an informant, usually the nearest relative, is essential if the patient is too disturbed, confused or uncooperative to give a full history. In other cases it often adds useful information too, especially on the premorbid personality and the extent to which the illness has disrupted the patient's life, but should only be done with the patient's consent.

Social Work Report

By talking to the patient, preferably at home, and interviewing (with the patient's agreement) relatives, friends, neighbours or workmates, a social worker can obtain additional information about the psychiatric history and any other relevant problems, for example those concerning marriage, family, work and finance. Though often useful, a social work report is no longer routine in most psychiatric units.

Clinical Psychology Report

Psychometric tests, measuring such parameters as intelligence, memory, perception, behaviour and personality, may be useful aids to assessment especially in patients with organic brain damage. Psychological tests which quantify the type and severity of impairments, and identify those abilities which still remain intact, are helpful in planning rehabilitation programmes, also provide a baseline for monitoring long-term progress. Psychometric testing is no longer routine in most psychiatric units, because clinical psychologists have become more concerned with therapy than with diagnostic assessment.

PHYSICAL INVESTIGATIONS

The aim of physical investigation is to find a treatable lesion and/or make an aetiological diagnosis.

"Routine" laboratory tests seldom yield abnormal results in young adult psychiatric patients, unless there are physical symptoms or signs or a history of alcohol misuse. Screening of younger patients who appear to be in good physical health is therefore not clearly cost-effective, although many units do in practice carry out blood tests on all new admissions and these reveal occasional cases of unsuspected organic disease, most commonly thyroid dysfunction in women.

Elderly patients, and patients of any age with symptoms or signs suggesting physical illness, do need investigation. Basic tests include blood count and erythrocyte sedimentation rate (ESR), urea and electrolytes, thyroid and liver function, urine testing for glucose, protein, cells and bacteria, and chest X-Ray (but skull X-Rays very seldom yield useful information). Other tests such as an EEG, brain scan, analysis of blood or urine for drugs, syphilis serology and HIV testing may be done if clinical indications exist. (Except in very special circumstances, HIV testing should not be carried out unless the patient gives informed consent, and receives both pre- and post-test counselling.)

The EEG

The electroencephalogram (EEG) records the pattern of electrical activity from various parts of the brain. The main types of activity are called alpha, beta, delta and theta. Most, but not all, patients with organic brain disorders show abnormalities on EEG. The main practical use of the EEG is in the diagnosis of epilepsy; for detecting focal brain lesions, CT or MRI scans are more helpful. Patients with untreated "functional" psychiatric illness usually have normal EEGs, but treatment with psychotropic drugs and ECT alters the pattern.

Brain Scans

- *CT* or *CAT* (computerised axial tomography) involves scanning from different angles using an X-Ray tube and detector system, and reconstruction of cross-sectional or coronal pictures to provide views of both the brain and the ventricular system.
- *MRI* (magnetic resonance imaging) or *NMR* (nuclear magnetic resonance) works by recording the response to radio waves applied to the body within a magnetic field. No radiation risk is involved. Clear pictures of both white and grey matter may be obtained from any desired angle. MRI is superior to CT for some purposes, but less widely available.
- *PET* (positron emission tomography) works by detecting local concentrations of radioisotopes, and provides information about function, for example glucose or oxygen consumption and activity of different neurotransmitters.
- *SPECT* (single photon emission computerised tomography) utilises nuclear radiotracers to localise different receptors.

PET and SPECT are only available in a few centres in Britain, and are likely to remain research tools for the foreseeable future.

EEGs and brain scans are only carried out if there is clinical reason to suspect neurological disorder.

FURTHER READING

Books

Hodges JR (1994) *Cognitive Assessment for Clinicians*. Oxford University Press: Oxford

Leff JP, Isaacs AD (1992) *Psychiatric Examination in Clinical Practice* (3rd edn). Blackwell Scientific Publications: Oxford

Royal College of Psychiatrists (1994). *Psychiatric Instruments and Rating Scales* (2nd edn). Royal College of Psychiatrists: London

Sims ACP (1987) *Symptoms in the Mind: an Introduction to Descriptive Psychopathology*. Baillière Tindall: London

Thompson C (ed) (1989) *The Instruments of Psychiatric Research*. Wiley: Chichester

Trzepacz PT, Baker RW (1993) *The Psychiatric Mental State Examination*. OUP: Oxford

Review Articles

David A, Blamire A, Breiter H (1994) Functional magnetic resonance imaging. *British Journal of Psychiatry* **164**: 2–6

Moseley I (1995) Imaging the adult brain. *Journal of Neurology, Neurosurgery and Psychiatry* **58**: 7–21

Snaith P (1991) Measurement in psychiatry. *British Journal of Psychiatry* **159**: 78–82

II
Clinical Syndromes

4
Schizophrenia

DEFINITION

Schizophrenia is a psychotic illness, which in its active phase entails delusions, hallucinations and disturbance of multiple mental processes. Many cases run a chronic course leaving residual psychiatric symptoms and impaired social functioning.

Schizophrenia is often considered the most serious of all psychiatric conditions. Its importance has been more widely appreciated by society in recent years, since patients who would once have spent their lives in mental hospitals are now receiving "community care".

FREQUENCY

- *Incidence*: 10–20 new cases per 100 000 population per year.
- *Prevalence*: 2–4 cases per 1000 population at one time.
- *Lifetime expectation*: 0.5–1%.

Both the incidence and the severity of schizophrenia appear to have declined in recent years.

EPIDEMIOLOGY

- *Age*: onset is usually in late adolescence or early adult life, though the paranoid form may begin in middle or old age. Mean age of onset is 28 for men and 33 for women.

- *Sex*: equal sex ratio.
- *Marital status*: single status is more common than in the general population (and patients' fertility is low).
- *Social class*: rates are highest in classes IV and V. This is the effect of "drift down the social scale" as a result of the illness, rather than a reflection of parents' social class.
- *Nationality*: rates are similar in most countries, but apparent differences result from variations in diagnostic criteria. Migrants have raised rates.

CAUSES

Many biological, psychological and social factors have been implicated. These varied aspects can be integrated through the concept of "neurodevelopmental disorder", which implies that subtle damage to brain structure and/or function, occurring from a variety of causes before birth or soon afterwards, sets up the vulnerability to schizophrenia. Clinical symptoms develop in early adult life if the vulnerable person is exposed to biological or psychosocial stress.

The main lines of investigation are as follows:

- *Genetics*: genetic predisposition to schizophrenia is proven. The observed inheritance pattern fits a polygenic model in some families and a single gene of incomplete penetrance in others. There is not yet consistent evidence to localise the gene(s) to specific chromosomes.

Lifetime expectation of developing schizophrenia among relatives of a patient with the condition is as follows:

Parent	6%
Sibling	10%
Child (one parent affected)	14%
Child (both parents affected)	46%

Twin studies show concordance rates to be:

Monozygotic	35–58%
Dizygotic	9–26%

Studies of twins reared apart, and of children adopted away from their schizophrenic parents, show only slightly lower rates, suggesting that the genetic contribution to aetiology is substantial.
- *Neurochemistry*: the "dopamine hypothesis" is the most widely accepted biochemical theory. Dopamine is a monoamine neurotransmitter, synthesised from L-tyrosine via L-dopa. Dopamine is concentrated in three parts of the brain: the nigrostriatal tract (dopamine depletion in this area causes Parkinsonism), the hypothalamus (where dopamine inhibits release of prolactin) and the mesolimbic system, where excess dopamine activity is believed to occur in schizophrenia. This could reflect an excess of dopamine itself, or deficiency of dopamine antagonists such as gamma-aminobutyric acid (GABA) and acetylcholine, or increased sensitivity of dopamine receptors. Evidence in support of this theory includes:
    - most antipsychotic drugs, effective in treating schizophrenia, block dopamine receptors (D2 type), and neuroleptic potency is directly proportional to receptor blocking potency
    - schizophrenic symptoms can be precipitated by drugs, such as amphetamines, which increase dopaminergic activity
    - postmortem studies on brains from schizophrenic patients have shown excess dopamine concentration in the limbic system
    - PET studies in living patients indicate an increase of D2 receptors in the mesolimbic area.
- *Macroscopic brain disease*: any kind of organic brain lesion may give rise to symptoms resembling schizophrenia. Even patients without gross brain disease often show minor neurological signs, or have abnormalities on EEG, brain scan or postmortem brain study. Findings include enlargement of the lateral ventricles, and lesions of the medial temporal lobe and hippocampus. These are thought to reflect abnormal brain development in early life, but degeneration at a later date might also contribute. In support of the importance of brain damage are clinical observations that schizophrenia is associated with:
    - *temporal lobe epilepsy* of the dominant hemisphere
    - *birth complications*
    - *winter birth*
    - *maternal viral infection* in pregnancy (though evidence for this is conflicting).
- Psychodynamic and social theories:
    - *personality*: in about 50% of patients, premorbid personality

has "schizoid" features such as social isolation and eccentricity, though this may represent a prodrome of the illness itself. Prospective cohort studies have shown that children who show such features have an increased risk of schizophrenia in later life

- *family dynamics*: abnormal family relationships are no longer believed to be a primary aetiological factor. If present, they are probably consequence rather than cause of the disease. However, patients living with critical, over-involved parents who show high levels of "expressed emotion" (EE) are known to be at increased risk of relapse
- *life events*: life event experience can trigger an acute episode.

CLINICAL FEATURES

Onset of schizophrenia may be sudden or gradual. Symptoms include abnormalities of thought, ideation (delusions), perception (hallucinations), emotion, volition, or motor behaviour.

- *Thought*:
  - *thought interference* includes *thought insertion* (a sensation that some outside agency is putting thoughts into one's mind), *thought withdrawal* (the opposite experience) and *thought broadcasting* (the belief that one's thoughts are being communicated to other people)
  - *thought block* is the abrupt complete cessation of a train of thought
  - *knight's move thinking* (asyndetic thinking, derailment of thought) is abrupt transition from one topic to another unrelated one
  - *concrete thought* is inability to appreciate abstract concepts, though some patients show the opposite tendency and assume symbolic meanings which are not intended
  - *poverty of thought* is one of the "negative" symptoms characteristic of the chronic stages of the illness.

Abnormalities of thought are reflected in *speech*, which may be vague and difficult to follow, include odd changes of topic, or be incomprehensibly bizarre. Some patients keep repeating the same words or phrases (verbigeration), use idiosyncratic words (neologisms), or speak in a jumble of words (word salad).

- *Delusions*: onset of schizophrenia may be preceded by *delusional mood* in which the patient feels perplexed because the environment seems subtly changed. This feeling may be suddenly followed by a *primary delusion* (*autochthonous delusion*), usually linked with an ordinary sense perception (*delusional perception*). For example, one patient saw a yellow car drive by and took this to mean that he was Christ reincarnated. Delusions are most often paranoid, but may be of any kind. A complex system of secondary delusions may be elaborated from the primary one.
- *Hallucinations*: most commonly auditory. Voices discussing the patient in the third person are characteristic but second person voices which talk to the patient are common too. The patient usually attributes voices to an external source. Somatic, tactile, visual, olfactory or gustatory hallucinations may also occur.
- *Emotion*: *blunting* (or *flattening*) *of affect* means that the patient shows minimal emotion. *Incongruity of affect* is emotion inappropriate to the circumstances. Extreme mood changes of elation, depression or rage may occur. Sustained *depressive symptoms* are found in at least 50% of patients on follow-up, and are probably part of the schizophrenic process, though they may also represent side-effects of antipsychotic drug treatment, or a response to realisation of having such a serious disease.
- *Volition*: *passivity feelings*, in which emotions or actions are felt to be controlled by an outside agent, may be present. Bizarre urges out of keeping with the previous personality may occur. Most patients lack initiative and drive regarding activities of daily life.
- *Motor behaviour*: abnormalities are prominent in the catatonic form of schizophrenia and include mannerisms, stereotypies, imitation of the speech and behaviour of others (echolalia and echopraxia), negativism, mutism, stupor, hyperactivity, and prolonged maintenance of strange postures (waxy flexibility).
- *Cognitive function*: the defects found in chronic cases are probably part of the disease process, though they may be exacerbated by institutionalisation and physical treatments. Memory and attention are particularly impaired.

Symptoms are sometimes divided into *positive*, such as delusions and hallucinations, and *negative*, such as poverty of thought and speech, lack of initiative, social withdrawal, slowness, unreliability and poor self-care. Positive symptoms are prominent during acute episodes, negative symptoms are characteristic of the chronic stage.

Case Example

A 23-year-old woman still lived with her parents. She had always been quieter than her siblings, who had all left home, and she worked as a clerk in her father's business. Very gradually over a two year period, she began to find her work more difficult, repeatedly checking and finding new tasks extremely stressful. Spending more and more time in her room, she became preoccupied with books of a religious nature, though she ceased attendance at church.

Her family consulted the GP, who felt unsure, particularly as he knew that the family were members of an unusual religious sect. Provisionally, he diagnosed an obsessive-compulsive disorder and discussed psychiatric referral, but patient and family declined. He advised clomipramine, but the prescription was never dispensed.

Over the following weeks, the young woman began to try to prevent her parents going to church. A crisis developed when she locked herself in her room, and her father broke down the door to find her worshipping naked at a makeshift altar equipped with artefacts from various religions. A psychiatrist visited as an emergency, and found her to be thought disordered, with various ill-formed delusions of a religious nature; he made a provisional diagnosis of a first episode of schizophrenia. She declined medication or admission to hospital. The GP and social worker agreed that compulsory admission was indicated, but the family withheld consent until the patient cut her wrists two days later.

She improved in hospital, with ongoing antipsychotic drug treatment, but her subsequent course included relapses which were felt to be at least partly due to the family's overinvolvement, in particular a persisting belief that her disorder required religious rather than medical treatment.

A more recent subdivision of symptoms describes three groups: reality distortion, disorganisation and psychomotor poverty.

Physical health in patients with schizophrenia may be impaired because of heavy smoking, unusual eating habits, excess fluid consumption leading to water intoxication, poor hygiene, lack of exercise, other forms of self-neglect, and the side-effects of antipsychotic drugs (Ch 23) on various body systems.

CLINICAL TYPES

The following summary, based on the ICD-10 classification, depends on the description of clinical syndromes. It is not known whether these represent truly distinct entities.

● *Paranoid schizophrenia* has delusions, often accompanied by hallucinations, as prominent symptoms. If there are few other symptoms, and the general personality is well preserved, the condition may be called *paraphrenia*. Paranoid schizophrenia usually develops later in life than the other types, and schizophrenic illness starting after middle age nearly always takes this form. It is commoner in women, and in those with impaired hearing. Genetic factors seem less important than for other types of schizophrenia. Some rare psychiatric symptoms in which isolated paranoid symptoms occur (Ch 8) overlap with paranoid schizophrenia.
● *Hebephrenic schizophrenia* (a term seldom used in clinical practice) has an acute onset and florid symptoms which usually include delusions and hallucinations, thought disorder, and affective changes.
● *Catatonic schizophrenia*, which is rare, has predominantly motor symptoms.
● *Simple schizophrenia* (another term now seldom used) is characterised by negative symptoms of gradual deterioration of the personality, with flattening of affect, withdrawal from reality, and loss of drive, resulting in a lifestyle of social isolation and self-neglect. Positive symptoms seldom occur, so it is debatable whether a diagnosis of schizophrenia is actually justified in such cases.
● *Residual schizophrenia* is the defect state which may remain following an acute episode. Positive symptoms have faded but negative symptoms, with blunting of affect and thought disorder, remain.

Related conditions include:

● *Schizotypal disorder*, in which there are chronic anomalies of behaviour, thought and affect resembling those of schizophrenia but not meeting definite criteria. It overlaps with schizoid and paranoid personality disorders (Ch 7). Older terms include *latent, borderline* and *pseudoneurotic* schizophrenia.
● *Delusional disorders* (Ch 8).
● *Acute and transient psychotic disorders.*
● *Schizo-affective psychosis*, in which manic or depressive (affective) symptoms co-exist with schizophrenic ones, and the illness follows a course of relapses and remissions.

DIAGNOSTIC CRITERIA

Present criteria are purely clinical and not fully satisfactory. Controversies about the diagnosis of schizophrenia include:

- Whether the term should be reserved for illnesses which result in permanent residual defects (*nuclear* or *process* schizophrenia) or also used for acute episodes (*schizophreniform reactions*) which may recover completely.
- Whether the different clinical types of "schizophrenia" are variants of the same disease process, or separate conditions.
- Whether cases without positive symptoms should be included.
- Whether there is a valid distinction between schizophrenia and the affective psychoses.

When Kraeplin described the condition in 1896 under the name *dementia praecox* he distinguished it from manic-depressive illness because of its worse prognosis. E Bleuler, who coined the term "schizophrenia" in 1911, considered the essential features were loosening of associations in thought, flattening or incongruity of affect, ambivalence and autism (withdrawal from reality) and some permanent defect in personality. As these symptoms cannot be precisely defined, widely differing concepts of "schizophrenia" developed in different centres; for example schizophrenia was diagnosed more readily in the USA than the UK until the introduction of stringent diagnostic criteria such as those in the DSM classifications.

In recent years there have been attempts to standardise the definition. A popular system in Britain is that of Schneider (1959) who postulated a set of *first rank symptoms*, any one of which would be diagnostic of schizophrenia in a patient without organic brain disease. They are:

- *Auditory hallucinations* in one of three forms: voices discussing the patient in the third person, voices making a running commentary on his actions, and voices repeating his thoughts aloud (*echo de la pensée*).
- Thought insertion, withdrawal or broadcasting (*thought interference*).
- *Bodily (somatic) feelings of influence.*
- *Passivity feelings.*
- *Delusional perception.*

Schneider's criteria are arbitrary, do not predict long-term outcome, and may occur in patients who have affective psychoses rather than schizophrenia.

Many other alternative sets of diagnostic criteria have been proposed. There is poor concordance between them. Further advances will probably come from research in molecular genetics and neurochemistry rather than from clinical observations.

DIFFERENTIAL DIAGNOSIS

- *Organic brain disease*, such as temporal lobe epilepsy.
- *Drug-induced psychosis*: LSD, amphetamines, cocaine, "magic mushrooms", MDMA ("ecstasy").
- *Affective psychosis*.
- *Obsessive-compulsive disorder*.
- *Personality disorder*.
- *Acute reactions to stress*, especially in adolescents.
- *Simulation* of mental illness: rare.

Some of these conditions may present as indistinguishable from schizophrenia, and the correct diagnosis can only be made after investigation of physical factors, a period of observation, especially if the episode was triggered by drug misuse, and/or a trial of antipsychotic treatment.

TREATMENT

- *Drugs* (Ch 23): antipsychotic drugs such as chlorpromazine and haloperidol are effective in controlling positive symptoms in about 90% of acute cases, and form the mainstay of treatment. Oral administration is usually suitable, but severely disturbed patients often need intramuscular doses to start with. Medication may need to be given for up to four weeks before improvement occurs.

Patients who have made a good recovery from a first episode of schizophrenia may be able to taper off their medication after a few months. Those who have persistent symptoms, or frequent relapses, are usually kept on medication indefinitely but as long-term therapy carries a high risk of side-effects, and wastes time and money if it is not necessary, it is worth gradually withdrawing drugs for medium-prognosis patients to see if relapse occurs or not. Patients must be observed frequently during and after drug withdrawal.

Long-term medication is usually given by intramuscular depot injections. This method improves compliance, since many schizophrenic patients cannot be relied upon to take tablets regularly. It also ensures that patients are seen regularly by a community nurse or GP.

Antidepressant drugs, and lithium, usually in conjunction with antipsychotics, may also be of value in long-term management of schizophrenia.

- *ECT* (Ch 24) is often effective, at least in the short term, for patients who have failed to respond to antipsychotic drugs, who have a depressive component to their illness, or show catatonic symptoms.
- *Psychological treatments* (Ch 22):
  - *family therapy* of a structured kind, including elements of education of patient and relatives about the illness and the reduction of high "expressed emotion" (EE), has been shown to improve outcome for those patients who live in the family home. Support for relatives, provided by mental health care professionals and/or self-help organisations, is important
  - *cognitive-behavioural therapy* appears to help some patients to cope with their delusions and hallucinations.

Psychodynamic psychotherapy is not usually considered appropriate for schizophrenia.

- *Social aspects* (Ch 26): many first episodes require inpatient treatment. Emergency admission, sometimes under the Mental Health Act 1983, is required for acutely disturbed patients. Others can be managed in the community. After acute symptoms are under control, many patients benefit from some months of rehabilitation including guidance in work, practical aspects of daily living, behavioural modification and social skills.

In the past, many patients spent the rest of their lives in the chronic wards of large mental hospitals, but such institutions are currently closing down. Most patients are now managed by community mental health teams working in collaboration with primary care. Hostels or group homes provide a suitable environment for those who cannot live independently or with their families, and day centres or sheltered workshops offer supervised activity. Some patients, however, live rough, or in unsupervised lodgings, either because no suitable accommodation can be found for them, or because they

---

Case Example

A single man in his 40s had, at the age of 27, been admitted to the County Asylum with an episode of acute schizophrenia, showing delusions and hallucinations, for example that white motor cars were emitting poisonous fumes and harmful rays. Although he made a prompt recovery from the acute symptoms, he had remained an inpatient until the closure of the institution was being planned in the late 1980s.

At this time, the patient had some residual "positive" symptoms, the severity of which depended on how well he was complying with his oral chlorpromazine treatment. However, he was much more handicapped by "negative" symptoms such as poor self-care and an inability to occupy himself.

Although he would rather have stayed in the old hospital, it was resolved to try to resettle him in the community. He was eventually discharged into a group home with three other patients and a resident carer, plus a community psychiatric nurse and attendance at a day centre. Shortly afterwards, he suffered an acute relapse of his vehicle-related symptoms and had to be admitted to the new local District General Hospital psychiatric unit. His first year in the group home was punctuated by similar episodes, until he was put on a depot antipsychotic.

Some years later, this man has settled well into his new home. Although far from perfect, his self-care is much better and he is also, after much encouragement from an occupational therapist and other staff, taking an interest in the garden. He now says that he prefers his present accommodation to the Asylum.

---

reject offers of help. They are easily lost to follow-up especially in inner-city areas and, in the absence of medical or social care, there is a serious risk of self-neglect, self-harm, and occasionally of violence to self or others. Use of the *Care Programme Approach* (Ch 26), in which high-priority cases are monitored through a register and each patient has a named key worker, should enable medical and social care to be coordinated and maintained.

PROGNOSIS

About 25% of patients make a good recovery from a first episode of schizophrenia. About 10% require long-term institutional care. The rest, while able to live relatively independently, continue to suffer chronic symptoms and may experience intermittent acute relapses.

Poor prognostic factors include a premorbid personality of schizoid type, with poor social adjustment; onset of illness early in life; gradual onset of illness without precipitating life stress; predominance of negative symptoms such as affective flattening; and delay between onset of symptoms and starting drug therapy.

Suicide, often occurring by a violent method and without warning, accounts for death in about 15% of patients.

FURTHER READING

Carpenter WT, Buchanan JW (1994) Medical progress: schizophrenia. *New England Journal of Medicine* **330**: 681–690

Chua SE, McKenna PJ (1995) Schizophrenia – a brain disease? A critical review of structural and functional cerebral abnormality in the disorder. *British Journal of Psychiatry* **166**: 563–582

Davies T (1994) Psychosocial factors and relapse of schizophrenia. *British Medical Journal* **309**: 353–354

Kingdon D, Turkington D, John C (1994) Cognitive behaviour therapy of schizophrenia. *British Journal of Psychiatry* **164**: 581–587

Owen M, McGuffin P (1992) The molecular genetics of schizophrenia. *British Medical Journal* **305**: 664–665

5
Mood Disorders: Depressive Illness and Mania

Mood disorders (*affective disorders*) include depressive illness and mania. These are episodic conditions, occurring only once or twice in a lifetime for some patients but recurring at frequent intervals for others, usually with good recovery in between episodes.

- *Bipolar affective disorder* (formerly called *manic depressive psychosis*): both depressive and manic episodes.
- *Unipolar affective disorder*: recurrent depressive episodes, without manic ones.

Patients with manic episodes only are very rare.

The milder forms of depression are also considered in this chapter. Anxiety disorders, though sometimes classed with mood disorders, will be considered with the neuroses (Ch 6).

FREQUENCY

Depressive illness is among the commonest of psychiatric conditions, but estimates of its frequency vary greatly, depending on the method of case-finding and the diagnostic criteria used. Community surveys suggest that at least 10% of people satisfy diagnostic criteria for depression at any one time, and more than 20% experience one or more episodes during their lifetime. The vast majority of cases do not present to doctors. Mania is at least ten times less frequent.

EPIDEMIOLOGY

- *Age*: affective episodes may occur at any age, including child-hood, but tend to become more frequent in later life.
- *Sex*: depressive illness is diagnosed twice as often in women, partly due to a genuine excess, and partly due to more frequent GP consultation rates leading to higher detection. Mania has an equal sex incidence.
- *Marital status*: for men, rates of depressive illness are lower in the married than in the single, widowed or divorced. For women, the protective effect of marriage is less marked. Young married women with children have high rates of depression; single women have low rates.
- *Social class and occupation*: community surveys find highest rates of depression among the lower socio-economic groups, but bipolar disorders referred to psychiatrists tend to come from the professional classes. People who work in the creative arts have higher rates of affective disorder than those working at equivalent level in scientific fields.
- *Residential area*: depression is more common in urban districts than rural ones.

CAUSES

- *Genetics*: genetic predisposition is proven, and exerts most influence for bipolar disease. The lifetime risk of illness in relatives of affected patients is:

First degree relative	10–20%
Monozygotic twin	50–70%
Dizygotic twin	15–30%

- *Neurochemistry*: brain concentrations of monoamine neurotransmitters, and/or sensitivity of their receptor sites, appear to be altered in affective disorders. Noradrenaline (NA) and/or 5-hydroxytryptamine (5-HT, serotonin) are implicated for depressive illness, dopamine for mania. Evidence for neurotransmitter involvement includes:
  - most drugs which are effective in treating depression increase the availability of NA and/or 5-HT in the brain
  - hypotensive drugs such as reserpine, which deplete brain monoamine concentrations, can cause depression

- antipsychotic drugs, which block dopamine receptors, have a therapeutic effect in mania
- plasma concentration of tryptophan, a precursor of 5-HT, and the concentration of 5-HT in platelets are reduced in some depressed patients
- cerebrospinal fluid (CSF) concentration of the amine metabolites 5-HIAA (5-hydroxyindole acetic acid), HVA (homovanillic acid), and MHGP (methoxy-hydroxy-phenylethylene glycol), also urine concentrations of MHGP, are reduced in some depressed patients
- postmortems on depressed patients who died by suicide show low concentrations of 5-HT and 5-HIAA in the brain itself.

Such studies are difficult because delicate measurements are involved; concentrations of amine metabolites may reflect changes in the rest of the body rather than the brain itself; and findings may be affected by diet, exercise and diurnal rhythms.

- *Hormones*:
    - cortisol secretion in some patients with severe depression is increased up to twice normal values. Diurnal variation in cortisol levels is altered, and dexamethasone administration fails to suppress cortisol production. The *dexamethasone suppression test* has been used as an aid to the diagnosis of depression but is too non-specific to be clinically useful
    - growth hormone release in response to insulin-induced hypoglycaemia, or in response to clonidine, is impaired in depression
    - TSH response to TRH is reduced in depression
    - in women, the occurrence of postpartum and premenstrual depression suggests sex hormone balance can affect mood.

- *Social stress*: depressed patients report more "life events", especially loss events, than general population controls during the few months before their illness onset. About 80% of depressive episodes appear to be precipitated by life event stress. Chronic social difficulties, lack of confiding relationships and absence of a supportive social network are important mediating factors. Life events can also precipitate manic episodes but appear less important for subsequent episodes than first ones.

- *Psychodynamic theories*: inadequate parenting in childhood has been implicated in hindering sound personality development, leaving the subject low in self-esteem and vulnerable to depression when experiencing a loss event in later life. Many research studies show a link between loss of the mother in childhood and depression in adulthood.

Another postulated mechanism is that depression results from an inability to express hostility and aggression, so that these emotions are directed inwardly to produce self-blame and guilt.

• *Behavioural and cognitive theories*: the *learned helplessness* model states that depression results from repeated failure to overcome problems by personal effort.

The *cognitive* model, first proposed by Beck and currently much favoured, states that depressed mood may result from, or be perpetuated by, a habit of negative thinking, interpreting all events in their worst possible light, and drawing generalised pessimistic conclusions from an isolated minor set-back.

• *Personality studies*: certain personality traits may predispose to affective disorder. Bipolar disorder tends to develop in those of cyclothymic personality. Mild depression in younger people tends to affect anxious or dependent personalities with poor tolerance of stress. Severe depressive illness in middle age tends to affect hardworking, conventional people with high standards and obsessional traits. There are frequent exceptions to these general rules, and it is important to appreciate that patients in the throes of a depressive or manic episode may give distorted accounts of their previous personalities.

CLINICAL FEATURES OF DEPRESSIVE ILLNESS

• *Psychological* symptoms include dysphoric mood in the form of misery, anxiety, guilt, pessimism or hopelessness. Irritability and hostility are prominent in some patients. Enjoyment is lost (anhedonia), and energy, interest, concentration, decision-making, efficiency and sexual drive are impaired. Not all patients are aware of feeling depressed.

Some patients are mentally and physically slowed down (*retarded depression*), and may progress to *depressive stupor*. In others the depression is mixed with anxiety and overactivity (*agitated depression*). Older patients may show marked intellectual impairment (*depressive pseudodementia*).

Suicide is always a risk, and the interview should include tactful inquiry about suicidal thoughts and plans ("how do you feel about the future?" "do you ever get so low that life doesn't seem worth living?" "do you ever think about harming yourself?").

Severely depressed patients may develop *delusions* and *hallucinations* (psychotic symptoms). Delusions reflect the depressive thought content and may have paranoid, nihilistic, or hypochondriacal themes; for example, that the patient's body is empty or rotting away inside. Hallucinations often consist of voices in the second person, criticising the patient or advocating suicide.

● *Somatic* (biological, vegetative, physical) symptoms are just as common as psychological ones and often form the presenting complaint when depressed patients consult in general practice. Sleep is nearly always disturbed. Some patients wake early and cannot go back to sleep. This *early morning waking* is often linked with *diurnal variation*, with mood lowest on waking, followed by a lifting of mood as the day goes on; both these symptoms are strongly suggestive of depressive illness. Other patients have difficulty in getting off to sleep, and a few sleep longer than usual but find their sleep unrefreshing. Appetite is usually reduced, with consequent weight loss. A few patients eat more, and gain weight. Other somatic symptoms include constipation, amenorrhea, impotence, pain in various sites including head, face and back, fatigue and general malaise.

TYPES OF DEPRESSIVE ILLNESS

The classification of depressive states is complex and controversial. The word "depression" covers a wide range of conditions, from transient unhappiness to life-threatening psychiatric illness.

ICD-10 subdivides depressive episodes as follows:

● *Mild* (with or without *somatic* symptoms).
● *Moderate* (with or without *somatic* symptoms).
● *Severe* (with or without *psychotic* symptoms).

Severe depression is characterised by pervasive depression of mood which has a different quality from ordinary sadness, cannot be expressed by tears even if the patient wants to cry, and is unrelated to external circumstances. Somatic symptoms (early morning waking, diurnal variation of mood, anorexia, weight loss) are often prominent, and psychotic features (delusions and/or hallucinations) may be present. "*Major depression*", a term from DSM, denotes a clearcut severe episode. Severe episodes usually respond best to physical methods of treatment (see below) rather than psychological therapies alone.

Case Example

A 22-year-old man was brought to the GP by his girlfriend, who complained that over the previous few weeks he had become increasingly "moody and withdrawn", and been drinking too much. The GP, who had known him for years, was struck by his gaunt and miserable appearance, but was nevertheless surprised when, after his partner left the consulting room, the patient broke down in tears. There was a clear history of depressed mood, loss of interest in things which he usually found pleasurable, poor sleep with terminal insomnia, poor appetite with weight loss, and inability to concentrate leading to problems at work.

The GP, noting a positive family history of bipolar affective disorder in the father, made a diagnosis of depressive illness. He prescribed lofepramine, and, with the patient's consent, involved the girlfriend in discussing the nature and prognosis of the illness.

After the consultation, the GP realised that he had not yet assessed suicidal risk, and decided to call on the patient on the way home.

Mild depression is more common, and the symptoms more like an exaggeration of ordinary unhappiness. Mood varies depending on external circumstances. Somatic symptoms are not prominent, and delusions and hallucinations do not occur. There may be marked tearfulness, anxiety, irritability, and difficulty getting to sleep.

Dysthymia is a chronic mild depression or unhappiness, which may overlap with personality disorder. Recognising this often helps to make a realistic prognosis.

Depressive psychosis (hallucinations and/or delusions present) and *depressive neurosis* are rather outdated terms for symptom clusters now believed to represent the extremes of a spectrum rather than two different conditions. They correspond roughly to "severe" and "mild" depression.

Case Example

A 44-year-old married man came to the attention of a junior hospital psychiatrist after taking an overdose in the context of marital breakdown. He described depressed mood, anhedonia and continuing suicidal ideation. Although he made a fairly rapid improvement sufficient to return to work, his symptoms only partially resolved. The psychiatrist tried a number of antidepressants and some cognitive therapy to little avail and, determined to explore all treatment options, was thinking of suggesting ECT or referral for dynamic psychotherapy.

His consultant suggested discussing the patient with his GP, who turned out to know him well. The GP felt that, although he had benefited from treatment to get over the acute episode of distress, he had been "back to normal" for some time. The patient had "always had rather a gloomy outlook, just like the rest of his family".

The patient was accordingly discharged back to the care of the GP with a diagnosis of dysthymic personality.

Endogenous and *reactive* depression is another rather outdated distinction based on whether or not a precipitating life stress predating the depressive episode can be identified. Most depressive episodes are at least in part "reactive", in which case resolving the external stress and/or helping the patient cope with it more constructively should certainly be part of management. But it is important to consider biological treatments if symptoms of severe depression are present, however understandable the cause. For example, drug treatment can be helpful for depressive illness following life events such as bereavement (Ch 6), or in medically ill patients (Ch 11) including those with terminal disease.

Seasonal affective disorder (SAD) is a condition in which depressed mood accompanied by lethargy, excess sleep, increased appetite and irritability recurs each winter. It was believed to respond exclusively to light treatment; however recent studies indicate it can be just as effectively managed with standard methods such as medication.

Masked depression describes cases presenting with somatic symptoms when the patient denies depressed mood and may even appear cheerful and smiling.

DIAGNOSIS OF DEPRESSIVE ILLNESS

Most episodes of depression are brief and mild, and dealt with by the patient's own resources, or talking with a relative or friend. Of those who do present to doctors, the vast majority are dealt with in primary care. However, many of the depressive episodes identified by researchers both in primary care and in general hospitals have not been diagnosed in clinical practice. Sometimes this is because the patient's complaints are physical ones. Also, when depressive illness follows an adverse life event or is associated with chronic social difficulties or medical illness, it is easily put down simply to understandable distress.

Depressed mood which seems unduly severe or prolonged in relation to its apparent cause, the presence of somatic symptoms, or prominent guilt, pessimism, anhedonia, suicidal thinking and low self-esteem all suggest depressive illness.

Rating Scales for Depression

Standardised rating scales exist to permit quantitative measurement of the severity of depressed mood. Their main use is in research work, for example comparing response to different treatments. They may be used clinically as screening instruments to help detect depression in high-risk populations, for example patients attending general hospitals.

Observer-rating scales include the *Hamilton* and *Montgomery–Asberg*.

Self-rating scales include the *Beck*, *Zung*, *Carroll*, *Wakefield*, *Leeds* and *HAD* (*Hospital Anxiety and Depression*) *Scales*.

CLINICAL FEATURES OF MANIA

Manic symptoms can be considered the opposite of depressive ones. Mood may swing rapidly between cheerfulness, irritability or aggression. Energy is increased, with overactivity, disinhibition, distractibility, reduced need for food and sleep, increased sexual interest and financial extravagance. This behaviour may have disastrous consequences for the patient and for others, leading for example to bankruptcy or marriage breakup. Thought and speech are copious (*pressure of speech*), often with rapid loose connections between one topic and the next (*flight of ideas*), rhymes, and puns. Thought content is usually grandiose or paranoid. Delusions and hallucinations, also with a grandiose or paranoid content, may develop.

Hypomania is a term for mild episodes without delusions or hallucinations.

Manic stupor is a rare form in which activity is greatly reduced despite elated mood and grandiose thought content.
Transient periods of depression, sometimes lasting only minutes at a time, occur during most manic illnesses. If the periods of depression are more prominent, the illness may be called a *mixed affective state*.

DIFFERENTIAL DIAGNOSIS OF MOOD DISORDERS

● *Medical conditions*: depression can be an integral part of the symptomatology of some medical conditions, including neurological disorders such as Parkinson's disease, dementia, multiple sclerosis; endocrine disorders such as hypothyroidism; and virus infections such as influenza.
Manic symptoms may be due to organic brain lesions especially in the frontal lobe; toxic confusional states; endocrine disorders such as thyrotoxicosis or Cushing's syndrome.
● *Drug reactions*: drugs which may precipitate depression include hypotensives, especially reserpine and methyldopa, corticosteroids and possibly sex hormones, L-Dopa, digitalis, certain cytotoxics, certain antimalarials, sulphonamides and antipsychotics.
Drugs which may precipitate mania include corticosteroids, antidepressants, L-Dopa, LSD and amphetamines.
● *Psychiatric conditions*: depressed mood often accompanies other psychiatric disorders. In elderly patients, distinguishing between depressive illness and dementia is a common dilemma, though sometimes both are present together. Both depressive and manic symptoms may occur in combination with symptoms of schizophrenia: schizoaffective disorder. Agitated depression, and mixed depressive/anxiety neurosis, are easily mistaken for pure anxiety states. Antisocial personality disorder may be confused with mania.

TREATMENT OF DEPRESSIVE ILLNESS

Most depressive episodes which present in general practice, provided they are recognised, can be successfully treated with a combination of brief counselling and antidepressant drugs. About 10% are
referred to psychiatrists and the majority of these are managed as
outpatients, but hospital admission may be required for patients
who are suicidal, or refusing food and drink. Compulsory admission
under the Mental Health Act 1983 may be required. The three broad
categories of treatment are antidepressant drugs, electroconvulsive
therapy (ECT) and psychological approaches. These can be used in
combination with each other.

● *Drugs* (Ch 23):
  − *tricyclic antidepressants* such as amitriptyline and imipramine
    are the standard first line of treatment for depressive illness,
    and probably the most effective drugs for severe depression.
    They are effective in about 70% of depressed patients
  − *specific serotonin reuptake inhibitors* (SSRIs) such as fluoxetine
    and paroxetine are now considered by some psychiatrists and
    many GPs to be the treatment of first choice, because they are
    safer in overdose than tricyclics and may have fewer side-
    effects. Others consider that SSRIs, which are more expensive, should be reserved for patients who cannot take
    tricyclics or have failed to respond to them
  − *monoamine oxidase inhibitors* (MAOIs) such as phenelzine and
    moclobemide are less often prescribed but sometimes dramatically effective when tricyclics have failed
  − *lithium* is mainly used in the prevention of recurrent affective
    disorder, but is also useful in an established depressive episode
    as adjunctive treatment to one of the antidepressants listed
    above.

A therapeutic trial of an antidepressant drug is often required when
diagnostic doubt exists. Frequent changes of drug are to be avoided,
and compliance needs checking. If and when an effective drug is
found, it should be continued at least six months after recovery to
reduce the risk of relapse, then gradually tapered off if the patient
remains well.

Case Example

A GP telephoned the psychiatrist who was responsible for her sector, and who did monthly clinics in her surgery, to discuss a 47-year-old woman who had been depressed for several months. Having benefited from a "recent course of amitriptyline" she had now relapsed, with a full depressive syndrome including low mood and biological symptoms such as loss of appetite and insomnia. The GP requested advice on "a change of antidepressant and/or admission".

On further discussion, it became clear that the patient had derived clear though partial benefit from amitriptyline 50 mg nocte; not appreciating the need for continuing medication, she had stopped the tablets when she began to feel better. The psychiatrist suggested that the patient had had the right treatment, but not enough of it for long enough, and advised restarting amitriptyline, and working up to a dose of 150 mg nocte. She offered to see the patient if needed, particularly if the GP was worried about suicide risk.

The GP was happy with this plan and, three weeks later, reported that the patient had restarted amitriptyline, but had been unable to go beyond 75 mg because of side-effects. Nevertheless, she was very much better. The psychiatrist strongly advised continuing medication until the patient was fully well and for six months thereafter, before cautiously considering reduction, and once again offered to see the patient for further education and advice about depression and its management.

• *Electroconvulsive therapy* (ECT) (Ch 24): ECT works faster than drugs and is therefore the treatment of choice for depressed patients who are suicidal, refusing food and drink, or severely distressed. ECT may work if drugs have failed. Patients whose depression is of life-threatening severity may require compulsory ECT under the Mental Health Act 1983 if they refuse this treatment or cannot give valid consent. ECT is effective in about 80% of patients with severe depression, and works better than drugs in psychotic cases with delusions or hallucinations. Mild depression seldom responds well to ECT. Prescribing an antidepressant alongside ECT is usually recommended.

- *Psychological methods* (Ch 22): a continuing supportive relationship with a trusted professional forms a valuable part of the treatment of all depressed patients.

Cognitive therapy, designed to modify habitual negative thinking patterns which contribute to depressed mood, is as effective as drug treatment in moderate or mild depression. *Interpersonal therapy*, focused on relationships with others, is also useful.

Psychodynamic psychotherapy may be indicated for prophylaxis of recurrent episodes of mild or moderate degree. During a severe depression a purely psychotherapeutic approach is not appropriate because it will not correct delusions or hallucinations, and may increase patients' feelings of guilt and unworthiness.

Social casework may be helpful if the patient's family relationships or life circumstances are disturbed, whether as cause or result of the illness.

Resistant depression: psychiatrists commonly see depressed patients who have not responded well to previous treatment, usually with medication. The following points need to be considered:

- Reassess the diagnosis, excluding underlying physical pathology.
- Are there social/family problems perpetuating the illness?
- Could cognitive therapy help habitual negative thinking patterns?
- Has the patient actually taken the medication?
- Have adequate doses have been given for long enough?
- Consider change of antidepressant class (tricyclic/MAOI/SSRI).
- Combination drug treatment (tricyclic + MAOI , or tricyclic + SSRI): infrequent specialist use only.
- Consider adding an adjuvant such as lithium and/or L-tryptophan to a tricyclic or SSRI (L-tryptophan is currently available on a named patient basis only).
- Consider psychosurgery (Ch 26) if all the above have failed.

TREATMENT OF MANIA

Hospital admission is desirable to prevent the adverse consequences of extravagance or disinhibited behaviour. Compulsory admission under the Mental Health Act 1983 may be required, since many manic patients have no insight into their illness. Neuroleptic drugs (Ch 23) are the first line of treatment. Lithium is an effective adjunct to neuroleptics, but does not act so quickly and would not be used alone except for mild cases.

If drugs fail to control a manic episode, a few ECT treatments (preferably given on a daily basis) usually succeed.

PROPHYLAXIS OF AFFECTIVE DISORDER

Prophylaxis in the form of long-term medication should be considered for patients whose lives are significantly disrupted by recurrent illness, say two or three episodes within five years.

For bipolar patients, *lithium* is an effective prophylactic, which prevents further episodes in 70–80% of cases. *Carbamazepine*, an anticonvulsant drug, is an alternative to lithium and the two drugs may be given in combination if neither has been successful on its own.

For unipolar patients, lithium is sometimes effective but antidepressant drugs are probably the best prophylaxis.

Psychological and social measures are also important. Interpersonal and cognitive-behavioural psychotherapies have preventive value. Many patients value the information and peer support available through voluntary organisations such as the Manic Depressive Fellowship.

Prognosis

From 70 to 90% of episodes of affective illness recover within a few months even without treatment. The rest become chronic and may last for years. Prognosis is better if treatment begins early during the episode.

Even if their first episode has recovered, 70–80% of patients will suffer one or more further attacks at some stage in their lives. Some patients become ill at regular intervals, or at the same time each year, usually spring or autumn. Bipolar patients may alternate between depressed and manic phases, or either type may be more frequent. The course for an individual patient is unpredictable. Around 10–15% will die by *suicide*.

FURTHER READING

Books

Paykel ES (ed) (1992) *Handbook of Affective Disorders* (2nd edn) Churchill Livingstone: Edinburgh

Review Articles

Farmer A, McGuffin P (1989) The classification of the depressions: contemporary confusion revisited. *British Journal of Psychiatry* **155**: 437–443

McGuffin P, Katz R (1989) The genetics of depression and manic-depressive disorder. *British Journal of Psychiatry* **155**: 294–304

Paykel ES (1989) Treatment of depression. The relevance of research for clinical practice. *British Journal of Psychiatry* **155**: 754–763

Paykel ES, Priest RG (1992) Recognition and management of depression in general practice. *British Medical Journal* **305**: 1198–1202

Piccinelli M, Wilkinson G (1994) Outcome of depression in psychiatric settings. *British Journal of Psychiatry* **164**: 297–304

Scott J (1988) Chronic depression. *British Journal of Psychiatry* **153**: 287–297

Scott J (1995) Prevention of depression; psychological and social measures. *Advances in Psychiatric Treatment* **1**: 94–101

Silverstone T, Romans-Clarkson S (1989) Bipolar affective disorder: causes and prevention of relapse. *British Journal of Psychiatry* **154**: 321–335

Storr A (1983) A psychotherapist looks at depression. *British Journal of Psychiatry* **143**: 431–435

Williams JMG (1984) Review article: cognitive-behaviour therapy for depression: problems and perspectives. *British Journal of Psychiatry* **145**: 254–262

WPA working group (1995) Dysthymia in clinical practice. *British Journal of Psychiatry* **166**: 174–183

6
Anxiety and Stress-related Disorders: The Neuroses

GENERAL CONCEPTS OF NEUROSIS

The term "neurosis" is still used by many psychiatrists, although discouraged in recent official classifications. Neurotic disorders can be considered as an exaggerated response to stress. In contrast to psychotic ones, neurotic patients are free from delusions and hallucinations, and usually retain insight.

Neurosis covers a range of common conditions including:

- *Generalised anxiety states*: continuous, unfocused anxiety.
- *Panic disorder*: episodes of acute, severe anxiety.
- *Specific phobias*: anxiety related to specific objects (e.g. spiders) or situations (e.g. agoraphobia, social phobia).
- *Obsessive-compulsive disorders*: anxiety related to obsessional thoughts or compulsive ritual behaviours.
- *Reactions to stress*: include adjustment reactions, post-traumatic stress disorder.

Anxiety is a feature of them all. Patients with a mixture of symptoms from several categories are sometimes said to have *general neurotic syndrome*.

Frequency

Community surveys suggest that 10–15% of the population are significantly affected by neurotic symptoms at any one time, and about 25% will suffer at some stage in their lifetime. However, an exact prevalence is impossible to determine because neurotic symptoms are not qualitatively different from normal experience, and prevalence will depend on the criteria used.

In medical settings, anxiety is even more common than in the general community. In primary care, anxiety states frequently co-exist with mild forms of depression, and it has been questioned whether there is any real distinction between the two. Anxiety, again often mixed with depression, is a significant problem for at least 25% of patients in general hospital wards and clinics.

Epidemiology

- *Age*: neuroses usually start in early adult life. Symptoms may continue into middle or old age, but a first episode in later life should raise suspicion of major depressive illness or organic disease.
- *Sex*: more common in women.

Causes

- *Genetics*: up to 20% of patients' first degree relatives are affected, usually by the same type of neurosis, but the familial tendency can be partly explained by the influence of home environment in early life.
- *Physiological and biochemical*:
  - overactivity of the sympathetic nervous system, and increased secretion of adrenaline/noradrenaline: these are closely related to the physical manifestations of anxiety. ACTH and cortisol are also raised
  - disordered activity of the limbic system of the brain, probably involving the inhibitory neurotransmitter gamma-amino-butyric acid (GABA); most anxiolytic drugs enhance GABA transmission
  - variation of symptoms with current physical status, for example female patients usually describe an exacerbation in the premenstrual phase, and symptoms may worsen or remit with virus infections.

- *Personality*: almost everybody has the capacity to undergo a neurotic reaction if under a sufficient degree of stress, but those of sensitive or insecure personality have a lower threshold for developing neurotic symptoms. Specific neurotic disorders tend to develop in subjects with the corresponding personality type, for example obsessive-compulsive disorders in those with obsessional traits.
- *Social stress*: most acute episodes appear to be precipitated by an adverse life experience. Long-term psychosocial problems such as marital difficulties often appear to contribute in chronic cases, though the direction of cause and effect may be uncertain.

Clinical Features

One or more of a wide range of mental and/or physical symptoms may be the presenting complaint.

- *Mental symptoms*:
    - apprehension/worry, either general ("free-floating") or focused
    - poor concentration
    - irritability
    - insomnia, usually of the "initial" type where the patient cannot get off to sleep but lies awake worrying.
- *Physical symptoms*:
    - cardiovascular symptoms such as tachycardia, palpitations
    - respiratory symptoms such as dyspnoea, chest pain
    - gastrointestinal symptoms such as dry mouth, nausea, anorexia, dysphagia, diarrhoea
    - muscle tension, including tension headache
    - fatigue
    - dizziness
    - sweating
    - tremor
    - frequency of micturition
    - flushing of the face and chest.

These physical symptoms can be explained by overactivity of the sympathetic nervous system, muscle tension and/or overbreathing. In many medical settings, both patient and doctor place more emphasis on the physical aspects than the mental ones, resulting in diagnostic confusion and unhelpful or even harmful treatment (see also Ch 9).

Patients are oversensitive to minor environmental changes, and difficulties in personal relationships are often associated.

Differential Diagnosis

- *Personality disorder*: personality disorder is a more persistent condition than neurosis, and tends to present with disturbance of behaviour and social adjustment whereas neurosis presents with symptoms. The distinction between "neurotic illness" and "neurotic personality" is clearcut in some patients, for example if an anxiety state develops in a previously well-adjusted subject following a stressful event, but in other cases both co-exist, as when a habitually nervous dependent subject has an episode of particularly intense distress.
- *Other psychiatric illness* such as major depression or alcoholism. If delusions or hallucinations are present, the main diagnosis must be a psychotic disorder, though the patient may have neurotic symptoms too.
- *Medical illness*, including systemic disorders such as thyrotoxicosis, and brain disorders such as temporal lobe epilepsy.
- *Substance misuse*: alcohol, caffeine (in tea, coffee or cola drinks) or other drugs.
- *Stress reactions* of normal degree. Anxiety is to be expected in certain situations and, if not excessive, may actually improve ability to cope.

Treatment

- *Drugs* (Ch 23):
  - *anxiolytic drugs* such as *benzodiazepines* are best taken only when symptoms actually occur, or shortly before the patient has to face an anxiety-provoking situation. Regular medication encourages tolerance and dependence, and for this reason benzodiazepines are recommended for short-term use only. However, for a small minority of chronic sufferers who have tried and failed with other treatments, long-term benzodiazepine treatment may form the best therapeutic option
  - *antidepressants*: sedative *tricyclics* such as dothiepin are often

given in anxiety disorders, though not generally licensed for this indication. Their full benefit may take several weeks but their useful hypnotic properties are immediate. Imipramine is effective in panic disorder, and *MAOIs* and *SSRIs* may be useful in many neurotic conditions

- *beta-blockers* such as propranolol help to control the physical symptoms of anxiety
- *antipsychotic* drugs in low dose.

- *Psychological treatments* (Ch 22):
  - *counselling* and *supportive psychotherapy* are generally beneficial. Explanation, particularly regarding the causes of physical symptoms, is important. Self-help leaflets, books and tapes are available. Simple lifestyle advice regarding exercise and diet, and avoidance of excess alcohol, caffeine and smoking may be relevant
  - *cognitive therapy* is designed to help patients put their symptoms into logical perspective and gain control over maladaptive patterns of thought
  - *behaviour therapy* is indicated for phobic anxiety, in which systematic desensitisation, modelling or flooding may be used; also for obsessive-compulsive disorders, using thought stopping, response prevention or flooding. Relaxation training and biofeedback are useful for control of physical symptoms, and social skills and assertiveness training for anxiety related to social interactions
  - *problem-solving* is a brief psychological technique shown to be effective for anxiety and depression in primary care
  - *dynamic psychotherapy*, individual or group, designed to explore the origins of the symptoms, improve personal relationships and change maladaptive attitudes, may be helpful for patients with insight and motivation. However, this treatment can raise anxiety and introspection and therefore makes some patients worse.

- *Social management*: environmental problems which are causing continued stress can sometimes be modified through social casework. Many common stresses, such as an unhappy marriage, job dissatisfaction and poverty, cannot be directly remedied but the patient can often be helped to deal with them more constructively.

- *Psychosurgery* (Ch 25): very occasionally used for patients with intractable anxiety or obsessive-compulsive symptoms, and effective in about 60%.

Prognosis

Some patients have a single brief episode which recovers completely (with or without treatment), some have recurrent episodes, and others are chronically incapacitated. Patients who develop an acute neurotic illness following a temporary stress, but had a sound premorbid personality, usually do better than those with longstanding symptoms, chronic stress or neurotic personality traits.

Chronic neurosis can give rise to severe handicap, and is associated with raised mortality from suicide and accidents, and from neurological, respiratory and cardiovascular disease. However, some patients improve when they reach later life.

Features of individual types of neurosis will now be described.

Case Example

A retired university lecturer clearly recalled a sudden attack of terror, shaking and sweating before going to his first dance when he was 16 years old. Several similar attacks occurred in later years at times of acute stress, such as taking exams. He also suffered from persistent anxiety symptoms in relation to more minor daily stressors, for example the night before giving a lecture to students he would often be woken by nightmares, and have several episodes of diarrhoea before work. Academically brilliant, he did well in his research career, but because of his fear of addressing large audiences and of travelling by air he did not pursue the prestigious professorship he might otherwise have achieved. A period of analytical psychotherapy in his 30s, undertaken following a divorce, helped him relate better to other people but his anxiety symptoms did not improve even after a successful remarriage. Over the years he gained temporary benefit from prescribed drugs, especially MAOIs, and from alcohol; but vigorous exercise helped as much as anything. He took early retirement at age 55, occupied himself with country walks and writing books, and felt calmer and happier than ever before.

GENERALISED ANXIETY DISORDER (ANXIETY STATE)

The prevalence of pure generalised anxiety disorder is about 3% of the population, and a further 8% have mixed anxiety and depressive disorder. Physical and/or mental symptoms of anxiety, as listed above, are present most of the time in the absence of real danger, and are "free-floating" rather than focused on any particular stimulus.

Most acute episodes seen in primary care are precipitated by obvious stressors, and respond to supportive interviews designed to help the patient to express and clarify feelings, and address any practical problems. If a specific treatment is required, a short (two to four weeks) course of benzodiazepines is safe and effective. Antidepressants are useful for the more chronic case, as are psychotherapy and relaxation training.

PANIC DISORDER

This diagnosis, made more frequently in the USA, has only been part of psychiatric classification for the past 20 years or so, and its status remains controversial. The condition is a chronic one which usually begins in young adult life.

Panic attacks are intermittent episodes of acute anxiety with marked physical symptoms: shortness of breath, dizziness or faintness, palpitations or tachycardia, trembling or shaking, choking, nausea, depersonalisation or derealisation, numbness or tingling, flushes or chills, chest pain. The patient may be terrified of dying or losing control. The attack may be misdiagnosed as a medical emergency such as a heart attack or epileptic fit.

First attacks often occur without apparent reason but later on, return to the situation in which previous episodes took place can precipitate further attacks and set up a pattern of avoidant behaviour (see agoraphobia below).

Cognitive-behavioural therapy, benzodiazepines and antidepressant drugs (including imipramine, phenelzine and SSRIs) are effective treatments.

AGORAPHOBIA

Agoraphobia, from New Latin and Greek, literally means "fear of the marketplace". Patients are afraid to visit shops or use public transport, especially if by themselves, and some are afraid to leave home at all. Panic attacks may occur in the feared situation, and some cases are secondary to panic disorder. Many patients are young married women of dependent personality ("housebound housewives"), whose husbands are overprotective and often have neurotic symptoms themselves. Behaviour therapy involving regular exposure to the feared situation is the best treatment. Antidepressant drugs may also help.

SOCIAL PHOBIA

Social phobias involve anxiety about being with other people, sometimes in a general sense, sometimes only in formal settings like parties or restaurants. Mild cases are very common. Behaviour therapy is the treatment of choice.

SIMPLE PHOBIAS (SPECIFIC PHOBIAS, MONOPHOBIAS)

Simple phobias are common in both childhood and adult life but only severe cases come to the attention of psychiatrists or psychologists. Anxiety is focused on a single phobic stimulus such as spiders, cats, air travel, vomiting. Sometimes the condition has an obvious explanation, as in the case of a young woman who was bitten by a dog, became preoccupied with a fear of dogs and altered her whole lifestyle to avoid possible contact with them; a "maladaptive learned response". Other phobias have no identifiable cause. Behaviour therapy is the treatment of choice, and consists of gradually increasing exposure to the feared phobic stimulus.

OBSESSIVE-COMPULSIVE DISORDERS

The patient feels a strong *obsession* to ruminate on a thought topic, and/or *compulsion* to carry out some practical action. The patient knows that these symptoms come from within the self, are inappropriate and should be under personal control, but attempts to resist them cause great anxiety and are usually not successful.

Common types of obsessional thinking include:

- fears of harming others (very rarely put into practice) or contracting a serious disease

- sexual or blasphemous thoughts which are abhorrent to the patient
- ruminations on insoluble problems in mathematics or philosophy.

Common types of compulsive rituals include:

- checking, for example that the door is locked or lights switched off
- washing, often carried out in order to allay fears of contamination or harm.

Patients may spend so much time on their rituals that normal daily activities are neglected. Compulsive hand-washers often develop skin lesions. The illness is particularly distressing because the patients are so well aware their symptoms are absurd.

Community surveys indicate that obsessive-compulsive disorder is present in 2–3% of the general population and, in contrast to other neurotic disorders, is equally common in both sexes.

Similar symptoms may occur as a sequel to encephalitis lethargica or other organic brain disease, and schizophrenic phenomena such as thought interference, passivity experiences and delusions may also cause diagnostic confusion. However, in organic and schizophrenic cases, insight and resistance are usually absent.

Behaviour therapy with exposure and response prevention, and antidepressants, especially those like clomipramine and SSRIs which act on 5-HT systems, are effective treatments. Psychosurgery is occasionally used, with good results.

CONVERSION AND DISSOCIATIVE DISORDERS

These disorders, formerly classified as "hysteria", tend to develop in response to severe stress. *Conversion* disorders (Ch 9) involve disturbance of physical function. *Dissociative* disorders involve disturbance of identity, memory or consciousness; types include psychogenic amnesia, fugue, and stupor. There is less agreement on the validity of other possible categories such as multiple personality disorder (Ch 7) and Ganser syndrome.

The *Ganser syndrome*, first described among prisoners and thought to be a form of malingering in many cases, consists of giving "approximate answers" to questions (Q: How many legs does a dog have?

A: Three), psychogenic physical symptoms, reports of hallucinations, and apparent clouding of consciousness.

Treatment is by psychotherapy rather than drugs.

POST-TRAUMATIC STRESS DISORDER (PTSD)

PTSD is described in survivors of major traumatic experiences, of a kind outside the normal range. Such experiences include large-scale disasters, whether natural or man-made, which cause multiple deaths and injuries (for example transport accidents, earthquakes); wartime combat; or individual trauma such as rape or domestic fire. Symptoms include:

- Persistent *re-experiencing of the trauma* through distressing night-mares or "flashbacks".
- *Avoidance of reminders* of the trauma, sometimes with actual amne-sia for the event. This may be accompanied by general feelings of detachment, loss of interest, inability to feel emotion, and "sur-vivor guilt".
- *Increased arousal*, for example insomnia, irritability, an exaggerated startle response.

The prevalence of PTSD in people exposed to extraordinarily distress-ing events ranges from 20–60% depending on the extent of involve-ment, the time elapsed, and individual vulnerability. Those who appear to have felt entirely out of control during the traumatic incident appear most at risk. The disorder may persist for years, with relapses at anniversaries. Many cases are complicated by alcohol misuse.

The mainstay of treatment is psychotherapy in which patients are encouraged to express their memories and feelings about the disaster in an individual or group setting. Antidepressant drugs may also help.

Early counselling for disaster survivors, often taking the form of "debriefing" where the subject is encouraged immediately to share experiences with others, is widely believed to help prevent PTSD though this is not proven.

ADJUSTMENT DISORDERS

Adjustment disorders are maladaptive reactions to psychosocial stress, lasting no more than about six months. Common symptoms include anxiety, depression, insomnia, behavioural changes and physical complaints. These symptoms, while falling short of a formal mental disorder, appear in excess of the "normal" reaction to the stressor concerned, and produce some impairment of occupational and social function. Counselling or social casework are usually considered more appropriate than drugs, though some patients do benefit from antidepressants or anxiolytics.

BEREAVEMENT

Grief following major bereavement has four classic phases:

- Shock, numbness, disbelief
- Protest, searching, pain
- Despair
- Acceptance

This model is a crude guide to a gradual process, which may take well over a year to complete. Similar reactions are found after other loss events such as death of a pet, breakup of a relationship, loss of a job, or mutilating surgery.

An abnormal grief reaction may be diagnosed if grieving is unduly prolonged, if grief cannot be expressed, or if there is denial that death has occurred. Bereavement may precipitate psychiatric illness, usually depression, or suicide in vulnerable people.

Abnormal grief reactions are more common if the deceased was young, if the death was sudden or violent, or if the bereaved person's relationship with the deceased was complicated by guilt or ambivalence.

Psychotherapy is often appropriate for abnormal grief reactions, for example the technique of "guided mourning" to help the patient acknowledge and grieve the death.

If severe depression develops after bereavement, drugs or ECT should be prescribed in the usual way.

CHRONIC FATIGUE SYNDROME

The diagnosis of *neurasthenia* was popular in the late nineteenth century and symptoms included fatigue after minimal effort, loss of interest, irritability, poor concentration and sleep disturbance. Similar syndromes have attracted great interest in recent years under new names such as *chronic fatigue syndrome*, *post-viral syndrome* and *myalgic encephalomyelitis* (ME). Some cases follow infection with the Epstein–Barr virus (which causes infectious mononucleosis or glandular fever) or other viral illnesses such as influenza, hepatitis, brucellosis, or encephalitis. In other cases no such infection can be identified, leading to controversy about whether chronic fatigue is primarily "organic" or "functional" in origin. Most cases probably represent the combination of the after-effects of a viral infection with a psychogenic reaction to stress in a person with obsessional and perfectionistic personality traits. Many patients have depressive symptoms, but it is not clear whether these are part of the syndrome itself, or a secondary reaction to it. Whatever the aetiology, psychosocial factors appear to be of prime importance in maintaining persistent symptoms and disability. Some patients, convinced that they are suffering from continuing viral illness, insist on continuing to rest, which causes loss of fitness and eventually makes fatigue worse. Others are willing to engage in a programme of gradually increasing activity, though often reluctant to consider that their problems may have a psychological dimension. Cognitive-behavioural treatment has been shown to be helpful.

FURTHER READING

Books

Sims A, Snaith RP (eds) (1988) *Anxiety in Clinical Practice*. Wiley: Chichester
Tyrer P (1989) *Classification of Neurosis*. Wiley: Chichester

Review Articles

Davidson A (1992) Drug therapy of post-traumatic stress disorder. *British Journal of Psychiatry* **160**: 309–314
Durham RC, Allan Y (1993) Psychological treatment of generalised anxiety disorder. *British Journal of Psychiatry* **163**: 19–26

Gelder MG (1986) Psychological treatments for anxiety disorders: a review. *Journal of the Royal Society of Medicine* **79**: 230–233

Gelder MG (1986) Panic attacks: new approaches to an old problem. *British Journal of Psychiatry* **149**: 346–352

Lader M (1994) Treatment of anxiety. *British Medical Journal* **309**: 321–324

Lynch S (1994) Chronic fatigue syndrome. *Advances in Psychiatric Treatment* **1**: 33–40

Marks IM (1986) Genetics of fear and anxiety disorders. *British Journal of Psychiatry* **149**: 406–418

Marks IM, O'Sullivan G (1988) Drugs and psychological treatments for agoraphobia/panic and obsessive-compulsive disorders: a review. *British Journal of Psychiatry* **153**: 650–658

Parkes CM (1985) Bereavement. *British Journal of Psychiatry* **146**: 11–17

Watson IPB, Hoffman L, Wilson GV (1988) The neuropsychiatry of post-traumatic stress disorder. *British Journal of Psychiatry* **152**: 164–173

7
Personality Disorders

DEFINITION

Personality disorders involve deeply ingrained maladaptive patterns of behaviour, which cause harm to the subject and/or to other people. These disorders are generally recognisable by the time of adolescence, and continue through most or all of adult life.

The older term "psychopathy" may be used for any personality disorder, but is usually reserved for the "antisocial" type.

CLASSIFICATION

Every personality is unique. The various types of personality disorder, as described below using ICD-10 terminology, overlap with each other and many individuals have traits characteristic of more than one type.

- *Paranoid*: suspicious, prone to the development of overvalued ideas including ideas of reference (Ch 8). Some subjects are sensitive and vulnerable, others aggressive about their rights. A small proportion develop a psychiatric illness with paranoid symptoms.
- *Schizoid*: shy, reserved, introspective, emotionally cold and shunning close relationships, often eccentric. A small proportion develop schizophrenia.

- *Dyssocial* (*antisocial, sociopathic, psychopathic*): showing repeated antisocial behaviour, not modified by experience or punishment. This type will be discussed in more detail below.
- *Impulsive*: emotionally unstable, prone to excessive outbursts of anger.
- *Histrionic*: prone to dramatisation and transient emotional displays, self-centred, craving for novelty.
- *Anankastic* (*obsessive-compulsive*): cautious, stubborn, conscientious, perfectionist, with high ethical standards. A small proportion develop a depressive illness or obsessive-compulsive neurosis.
- *Anxious* (*avoidant*): timid, cautious, lacking the energy and resilience to cope with minor stress.
- *Dependent*: compliant, passive, lacking in vigour.

The DSM-IV classification of the American Psychiatric Association describes some other categories, including:

- *Schizotypal*: includes avoidance of close relationships, eccentricities of cognition, perception and behaviour (for example "magical thinking"), and paranoid features. This may be related to schizophrenia.
- *Borderline*: characterised by impulsivity, variable mood, unstable relationships, self-damaging behaviour and uncertainty about personal identity.

Other personality types (not necessarily disorders) are described in clinical practice. For example the concept of *affective personality* would include the *depressive* type (always gloomy), the *hyperthymic* type (always elated) and the *cyclothymic* type (alternating between depression and elation). *Multiple personality* is a rare condition of dubious validity: it seems to develop in vulnerable individuals, encouraged by the interest and attention which the concept excites. *Sexual deviations* (Ch 17) may be considered as variants of personality.

DIFFERENTIAL DIAGNOSIS

- *"Normal" personality*: there is no fixed dividing line between the normal and disordered personality. Many of the personality traits mentioned above are only disadvantageous if present to extremes. Mild degrees may carry benefits in the right setting; for example, an anankastic personality may do well as a librarian, and a histrionic personality in the entertainment world. Personality disorder should only be diagnosed if the personality traits consistently impair well-being, personal relationships or work, or lead to dependence on drugs or alcohol.

● *Psychiatric illness*: personality disorders are relatively permanent conditions, whereas psychiatric illnesses involve a potentially reversible change from the patient's usual function. Personality disorders primarily entail abnormal behaviour, whereas psychiatric illnesses primarily entail mental symptoms. The distinction between personality disorder and psychiatric illness can be difficult, however, because:

– the same patient may have both
– personality disorders may only be obvious during times of stress
– patients are often unable to describe the difference between their current symptoms and their usual personalities.

An account from an informant, and long-term observation, usually resolve the issue.

● *Organic brain disease* often causes personality change.

TREATMENT

By definition, personality disorders involve persistent characteristics which cannot easily or quickly be eradicated. However, it is wrong to

---

Case Example

A woman in her mid-20s had always privately engaged in self-injurious behaviour. Following a divorce, she took overdoses and cut herself much more frequently, at least once a week. Repeated assessments failed to indicate any mental illness. Antidepressant medication had been tried without improvement; admission to acute psychiatric wards seemed to be associated with a worsening of her behaviour. She was admitted to a therapeutic community where self-harm was against the rules and would lead to discharge. Although she was apparently reluctant to address her psychological problems in the daily group sessions, her behaviour became much less troublesome during the year of her membership. It did return after she left, but remained at a comparatively low level. The cost of the treatment was less than that of the care she would have otherwise required.

assume that all these patients are untreatable: it may well be possible to contain or even modify undesirable personality traits and their ill-effects.

Psychotherapy aiming towards greater insight and improved behaviour patterns benefits some cases.

Drug treatment is sometimes helpful, in which case it usually needs to be continued on a long-term basis. Antidepressants (MAOIs or SSRIs rather than tricyclics), low-dose antipsychotics (sometimes given in depot form), and mood stabilisers (lithium or carbamazepine) have been successfully used. Drugs with a high potential for dependence, such as benzodiazepines, are best avoided in these patients.

PROGNOSIS

Long-term follow-up studies indicate a wide range of outcomes. Some patients improve considerably over time, whereas in other cases the features of disorder become even more deeply ingrained, and the risk of suicide is raised.

SOCIOPATHIC (DYSSOCIAL) PERSONALITY DISORDER

The Mental Health Act 1983 (using the older term *psychopathic disorder*) gives this definition: "A persistent disorder or disability of mind (whether or not including significant impairment of intelligence) which results in abnormally aggressive or seriously irresponsible conduct on the part of the person concerned."

Causes

- *Genetic predisposition* is suggested by adoption studies.
- *Brain damage*, usually dating from early life, is present in some cases and the EEG may show an immature pattern. Temporal lobe lesions may be especially implicated.
- *A disturbed upbringing* is often described, suggesting the condition may partly result from lack of guidance in childhood regarding acceptable behaviour.

Clinical Features

Sociopaths, most of whom are male, consistently behave in ways which are unacceptable to their culture and damaging to themselves, but seem unable to learn from experience. They seek immediate pleasures without considering the long-term consequences, and are unable to make lasting relationships with others, though some possess great superficial charm and are skilled in casual contacts. Subjects often report frequent changes of job, frequent moves of residence, and multiple sexual partners, and are living under stress of their own making. They often become depressed at such times, and/or experience transient delusions or hallucinations. Drug or alcohol misuse and criminal behaviour are frequent. "Inadequate", "aggressive" and "creative" types have been described. Many prison inmates have sociopathic traits.

Differential Diagnosis

- *Psychiatric illness*, especially hypomania and schizophrenia.
- *Organic brain disease*, especially frontal and temporal lobe lesions.
- *Drug-induced states*, especially amphetamines or LSD.

Treatment

There is no firm evidence that psychiatric treatment is helpful, but the Mental Health Act 1983 permits compulsory admission if it is considered likely that treatment will "alleviate or prevent deterioration of the condition", and many psychopaths are admitted to regional secure units under the Act.

The most effective management is thought to be psychotherapy in a group composed of other sociopaths. Therapeutic communities for this purpose include those at the Henderson Hospital, Broadmoor Hospital and Grendon Underwood Prison. Individual psychotherapy is seldom successful as patients are often manipulative, and unreliable in attendance.

Lithium and/or long-acting depot antipsychotics are often helpful in controlling aggression and mood swings. Patients with a temporal lobe abnormality may benefit from an anticonvulsant such as carbamazepine. Drugs should be prescribed with caution since there is a risk of overdose, dependence or abuse.

Prognosis

Flagrant antisocial behaviour usually diminishes with age, but problems with relationships continue. About 5% commit suicide.

See also Ch 21 on Forensic Psychiatry.

FURTHER READING

Blackburn R (1988) On moral judgements and personality disorders. The myth of psychopathic personality revisited. *British Journal of Psychiatry* **153**: 505–512

Piper A (1994) Multiple personality disorder. *British Journal of Psychiatry* **164**: 600–612

Stein G (1992) Drug treatment of the personality disorders. *British Journal of Psychiatry* **161**: 167–184

Stone MH (1983) Long-term outcome in personality disorders. *British Journal of Psychiatry* **162**: 299–313

Tyrer P, Casey P, Ferguson B (1991) Personality disorder in perspective. *British Journal of Psychiatry* **159**: 463–471

8
Paranoid States and Rare Named Syndromes

DEFINITION AND PSYCHOPATHOLOGY

Paranoid states involve distorted attitudes and beliefs, often concerning persecution. For practical purposes, the important distinction is whether the beliefs are *delusions* or *overvalued ideas*.

- *Delusions*: firmly held, incorrigible false beliefs, which are inappropriate for the person's racial, cultural, social and educational background. Delusions indicate psychotic illness or organic brain disease.
- *Overvalued ideas*: strongly held beliefs which are not so incorrect or unshakeable as to amount to delusions. Overvalued ideas and ideas of reference (see below) may be present in many psychiatric conditions including personality disorder, neurosis and psychosis, however they do not necessarily indicate psychiatric illness. The patient may retain some insight, realising that the ideas are unusual or could be mistaken.

Delusions may take on the status of overvalued ideas (become "less fixed") during the recovery from a psychotic illness, and vice versa during the prodrome to such an illness.

Both delusions and overvalued ideas may be classified according to content. The main types, with an example for each, are as follows:

- *persecutory (paranoid)*: "my neighbours are sending poisonous rays into my home"

- *of reference*: "people on the radio are talking about me"
- *grandiose*: "I have the power to cure every patient in this hospital"
- *of guilt*: "my evil thoughts caused the famine in Africa"
- *nihilistic*: "my mind is empty and can never work again"
- *erotic*: "the Prime Minister has made secret plans to marry me"
- *of jealousy*: "my husband singing that song proves he's having an affair"
- *somatic (bodily)*: "I am pregnant" (a belief held by a 70-year-old woman)
- *religious*: "The Devil is controlling my mind"

Some of these beliefs are so bizarre that they are obviously delusions; for others, it would be necessary to know more about the person's circumstances and cultural background before labelling them as such.

PREDISPOSING FACTORS

- *Paranoid personality characteristics*: paranoid personalities (Ch 7) are abnormally sensitive, conscious of their own rights, tend to see other people's behaviour as hostile, and are prone to develop ideas of reference. Overvalued ideas have often been present throughout adult life and influenced choice of lifestyle, for example living alone with minimal social contacts. The personality disorder may not present medically, but would colour the presentation of a superimposed mental illness, for example a paranoid person who became depressed might lack trust towards doctors or suspect that medication was poisonous.
- *Deafness*, and other forms of sensory deprivation.
- *Social isolation*.
- *Immigrant status*.

DIFFERENTIAL DIAGNOSIS OF PARANOID STATES

Paranoid symptoms are found in many of the common psychiatric conditions described elsewhere in this book, including *paranoid schizophrenia* (Ch 4), *affective disorders* (depressive illness and mania) (Ch 5), *drug and alcohol misuse* (Chs 12 & 13), the *dementias* (Ch 10). The following list describes some other syndromes in which paranoid symptoms are a primary feature.

● *Persistent delusional disorder* (older terms include *paranoid psychosis, paraphrenia, paranoia*): delusions are present, but in contrast to paranoid schizophrenia there are usually no hallucinations, the rest of the personality is preserved, and onset is in later life. The majority of patients have a paranoid premorbid personality, and interviews with informants may be essential to sort out whether the symptoms are new (an illness has developed), or whether they have always been present (personality) and have come to light for other reasons.

● *Acute paranoid reaction*: a transient condition provoked by stress.

● *Induced delusional disorder (folie à deux)*: a rare condition in which the same persecutory delusions are shared by two people, or sometimes several people, who live in close contact and are often genetically related. The "principal" who initiates the delusions suffers from schizophrenia or other mental illness. The "associate" who copies the delusions often has a dependent personality and low intelligence, and usually gives up the delusions if separated from the principal.

● *Morbid jealousy (pathological jealousy, Othello syndrome)*: patients, usually men, are deluded that their sexual partners are unfaithful. Morbid jealousy is often part of another syndrome: paranoid schizophrenia, depressive illness, organic brain syndrome, or alcoholism. Many patients have sexual dysfunction and/or poor personality adjustment. About 5% show homicidal behaviour, and lesser degrees of violence are even more common, so morbid jealousy is an important condition despite being rare. A formal assessment of dangerousness (Ch 21) must be made in such cases, and appropriate action such as referral to a forensic psychiatrist considered. Antipsychotic drugs, cognitive-behavioural therapy, and separation from the partner may help.

● *Erotomania (de Clerambault's syndrome)*: the patient, usually a woman, has the delusion that another person, usually a man of higher social status, is in love with her. This syndrome is often secondary to schizophrenia.

● *Capgras syndrome (illusion des sosies)*: the delusion that one or more close relatives have been replaced by a double. This syndrome is usually secondary to schizophrenia or organic brain disease.

● *Fregoli syndrome*: a rare delusion that a certain person, usually a persecutor, is psychologically present in the bodies of familiar people. Most cases are secondary to schizophrenia or organic brain disease.

Paranoid disorders with a somatic content are considered in Ch 9.

MANAGEMENT

Establishing a trusting relationship with the patient, though not always easy, is of prime importance in the treatment of paranoid states.

Objective information about the social setting and cultural background must be sought. Some "paranoid delusions" are based on genuine persecution, and some "religious delusions" could be viewed as spiritual experiences rather than a manifestation of mental illness.

A psychotherapeutic approach is often suitable for milder cases, but if delusions are present, an antipsychotic drug such as trifluoperazine or pimozide is indicated. Some patients are reluctant to take medication because they suspect it is poisoned, or insist they are not ill. Compulsory detention and treatment under the Mental Health Act 1983 may be necessary if there is disturbed or violent behaviour.

CULTURE-BOUND SYNDROMES

These conditions, confined to particular cultures, are conveniently mentioned here although it may not be strictly correct to class all of them as "paranoid states". Examples are:

- *Amok*: an acute confusional state occurring in Malaysian men, leading to murder and/or suicide.
- *Latah*: echolalia and echopraxia, in Malaysian women.
- *Koro*: panic caused by fear that the penis is disappearing, in young Chinese men.
- *Dhat*: complaints of losing semen in the urine, in young Indian men.

These rare syndromes are of academic interest rather than practical importance.

FURTHER READING

Books

Enoch MD, Trethowan WH (1991) *Uncommon Psychiatric Syndromes* (3rd edn). Butterworth Heinemann: Oxford

Review Articles

Gannon MA, Wrigley M (1995) Late paraphrenia. *British Journal of Hospital Medicine* **53**: 128–130

McKenna PJ (1984) Disorders with overvalued ideas. *British Journal of Psychiatry* **145**: 579–585

Todd J, Dewhurst K, Wallis G (1981) The syndrome of Capgras. *British Journal of Psychiatry* **139**: 319–327

9

Somatic Presentations of Psychiatric Disorder

Somatic (physical, bodily, biological, vegetative) complaints form part of the symptom pattern in all the common primary psychiatric disorders. Somatic presentations arise because emotional problems carry a stigma in patients' family or cultural setting and/or because patients genuinely perceive the bodily symptoms as predominant. Many psychiatrically ill patients, perhaps especially those from ethnic minorities, first present to their doctors with somatic complaints.

These patients are often referred to medical or surgical outpatient clinics because the psychological background is unrecognised. This can result in a long series of unhelpful, and expensive, hospital investigations and treatments.

Sometimes somatic symptoms have a demonstrable physiological basis, sometimes they seem to result from misinterpretation of ordinary bodily sensations. Such misinterpretation may be based on past experience of physical disease in other people or the patients themselves.

DIAGNOSTIC CATEGORIES

Classification and terminology for these disorders are complex, and vary substantially between ICD and DSM. The following summary is based on UK clinical practice. The syndromes may be primary, or secondary to another mental disorder in which case diagnosis and management would be guided by that of the underlying condition.

Psychiatric conditions in which somatic complaints are particularly important include:

• *Depressive illness* (Ch 5): often associated with anorexia, weight loss, constipation, tiredness and pain. Because of their pessimistic and hopeless cognitions, depressed patients may attribute these symptoms to physical disease of a serious and/or stigmatised kind, such as cancer or AIDS. Those with psychotic depression may develop full-blown delusions of having incurable illness.

• *Anxiety states* (Ch 6): autonomic overarousal, heightened muscle tension and overbreathing can produce a wide range of bodily symptoms. Anxious patients may attribute these symptoms to serious physical disease, for example they fear a heart attack if they experience palpitations.

• *Schizophrenia*, and *delusional disorders* (Ch 4): somatic delusions and hallucinations may occur in schizophrenia and are sometimes bizarre, for example a belief that the internal organs are upsidedown. Rare related conditions are characterised by fixed somatic delusions, for example patients with *monosymptomatic hypochondriacal psychosis* might believe that their skin is infested with parasites or their bodies emit a foul smell.

• *Somatisation disorder* (*Briquet's syndrome*): patients repeatedly consult their doctors about a variety of physical symptoms, in different body systems, for which no organic cause can be found. The disorder is a chronic one, which fluctuates over a period of several years, usually beginning in early adult life and affecting women more often than men. Most patients have severe social or interpersonal problems, and some are dependent on prescribed medication. Alcoholism and psychopathy occur to excess in male relatives of these patients.

• *Hypochondriasis*: this involves an unwarranted fear, or belief, of having one or more serious physical diseases (in contrast to somatisation where the patient tends to concentrate on the symptoms themselves). The fears and beliefs persist despite negative medical tests, but are not of delusional intensity. The syndrome is equally common in both sexes, usually starts in young adult life and follows a chronic course, indeed in many cases it is often best regarded as a personality trait. It is compatible with a normal level of psychosocial functioning.

- *Dysmorphophobia*: patients are preoccupied with a defect of appearance, for example a misshapen nose, which other people consider trivial. They often seek plastic surgery and in some cases this is helpful, but other patients remain dissatisfied even after repeated surgical revisions. In contrast with monosymptomatic hypochondriacal psychosis, the beliefs of dysmorphophobia are not of delusional intensity.

- *Psychogenic pain*: persistent severe pain, which cannot be explained by a physical disorder, and may be inconsistent with the anatomical distribution of the nervous system, but often seems to be associated with emotional conflicts or psychosocial problems. Some cases of neuralgia and headache fall into this category. First-line treatment is with antidepressant medication, which may be helpful even if a depressive syndrome cannot clearly be identified.

- *Conversion and dissociative disorders* (formerly called *hysteria*): *conversion disorder* is the current term for syndromes in which physical symptoms such as paralysis of a limb, blindness or fits, which cannot be explained medically, develop in stressful circumstances. Such symptoms appear to express an emotional conflict or need, and may bear some symbolic relationship to the nature of the stress. For example, one student developed a paralysed right hand the day before a written exam. The symptoms often appear to bring advantages for the patient: "primary gain" of keeping psychological stress at bay, and "secondary gain" of attracting sympathy and support or avoiding unwelcome obligations.

Most cases seen today tend to resolve quickly, though may recur under repeated stress. Florid cases, with severe features such as chronicity and unconcern about the symptoms ("la belle indifférence") are rare in modern Western society. Civilian cases tend to occur in women, but male cases are encountered in military settings during wartime. Epidemic forms occur, for example fainting at pop festivals, though other factors such as fatigue, infection, lack of food or drug misuse may contribute in such settings.

Dissociative disorder refers to a similar presentation with psychological symptoms, such as psychogenic amnesia or fugue.

- *Factitious disorder* (*Munchausen's syndrome*): patients, usually male, contrive repeated hospital admissions by fabricating acute physical symptoms such as bleeding or acute abdominal pain. They usually give a dramatic history under a false name. They may submit to

unpleasant investigations, or even to surgery, before suddenly discharging themselves and travelling to another hospital to repeat a similar performance.
- *Chronic fatigue syndrome*: see Ch 5.

MANAGEMENT

- *Excluding organic disease*: a minority of "somatising" patients referred to psychiatrists have a genuine physical illness which has been missed. The initial evaluation should always include making sure, preferably by personal discussion with the referring doctor, that appropriate physical assessments have been done. Some psychiatrists favour carrying out a physical examination themselves. If no evidence of organic disease has been found, the patient should be firmly reassured at the outset, but repeated reassurance is unhelpful. Following this, the psychiatrist often contracts with the patient that any requests for more sophisticated tests and second opinions should be addressed to the referring doctor, as patients may otherwise use this as a means of avoiding underlying psychological issues.
- *General approach*: somatising patients need tactful handling. Some are reluctant to consider a psychological aspect to their condition, are on bad terms with their doctors (the term "heartsink patient" has been applied to chronic somatisers in general practice) and angry if psychiatric referral is broached. Others welcome an opportunity to discuss the psychosocial background to their symptoms. If several healthcare professionals are involved it is important for them to cooperate with each other, to ensure a consistent policy.

A key point is that most of these disorders are to be coped with over long periods, rather than cured. The vast majority will be cared for by the primary healthcare team, and a GP who has known a patient for many years will often be able to identify lifelong hypochondriacal tendencies, and so contain an increase in symptoms and consultations at times of stress without needless interventions.

Case Example

A 27-year-old woman had been looked after by one GP through-out her life. Her parents had separated, her father being an alco-holic, and there was some suggestion that she had been sexually abused by her stepfather. She herself tended to form abusive rela-tionships with a succession of violent males, her main outlet being frequent consultations with her doctor with bitter complaints of symptoms in a variety of body systems. Although the GP viewed her as one of her "heartsink" patients, and never felt that she was achieving much progress, she managed to contain her with only infrequent symptomatic treatments and simple investigations.

While her usual GP was on holiday she consulted a locum, com-plaining of pelvic pain and in great distress. She was referred to the local gynaecologist. At the hospital, where she saw a succession of junior doctors, various medications were tried to no effect and eventually a hysterectomy was performed. The patient then com-plained that her pain had actually got worse. A psychiatric referral followed, and a diagnosis of somatisation disorder was made, but the patient was entirely unwilling to engage in any form of psycho-logical treatment and spoke of suing the gynaecologist.

- *Underlying psychiatric disorders* must be treated. For example, somatic delusions in psychotic depression often disappear following successful treatment of the depressive illness.
- *Specific psychological interventions*: it is important to explain the symptoms to the patient, not belittling them as trivial or unreal, but introducing the idea of mind–body interactions, for example by explaining the physiology of anxiety, or by pointing out time links between psychological stress and onset of symptoms. Giving positive suggestions that improvement is likely to occur with time is probably helpful. Specific therapy with a cognitive-behavioural approach (Ch 22) may enable patients to view their symptoms in a more logical way, and gain greater control over them. In other cases, a psycho-dynamic approach to the conflicts underlying the physical complaint is helpful.
- *Psychotropic drugs*: antidepressant drugs are sometimes effective for somatic complaints including pain, even if the patient is not overtly depressed, and neuroleptic drugs such as trifluoperazine or pimozide may control somatic delusions and hallucinations.

Case Example

A man of 48 was made redundant from an unskilled factory job, and could not find further work. He started to suffer severe headaches, and consulted his general practitioner several times. The GP's impression of a depressive component was vehemently rejected by the patient, and there seemed no alternative to neurology referral. Whilst waiting for outpatient consultation, the patient's pain became incapacitating over a weekend and he was admitted as an emergency. During a two week admission, he had extensive investigations, all of which were normal, and continued to refuse the ward staff's efforts to encourage him to talk about his apparent emotional problems. He was discharged with a diagnosis of "tension headache, ? depressed" on amitriptyline 50 mg nocte, in the belief that this drug was purely an analgesic. He continued to suffer headaches, and to decline more intensive psychiatric input. In follow-up, he never regained full physical or psychological health, though it was clear that he was rather better when taking amitriptyline than when not.

PROGNOSIS

Follow-up of patients with medically unexplained somatic symptoms shows that about one-third are found to have a medical diagnosis, one-third a psychiatric diagnosis, and one-third remain unexplained.

FURTHER READING

Bass C, Benjamin S (1993) The management of chronic somatisation. *British Journal of Psychiatry* **162**: 472–480

Creed F, Guthrie E (1993) Techniques for interviewing the somatising patient. *British Journal of Psychiatry* **162**: 467–471

Lloyd GG (1989) Somatisation: a psychiatrist's perspective. *Journal of Psychosomatic Research* **33**: 665–670

Mayou R (1991) Medically unexplained physical symptoms. *British Medical Journal* **303**: 534–535

Murphy M (1989) Somatisation: embodying the problem. *British Medical Journal* **298**: 1331–1332

Tyrer S (1992) Psychiatric assessment of chronic pain. *British Journal of Psychiatry* **160**: 733–741

10
Organic Brain Syndromes

Organic brain syndromes are conditions in which psychiatric symptoms result primarily from a biological disorder affecting brain function. This underlying biological disorder may involve structural cerebral pathology and/or metabolic disturbance. The patient's psychological reaction to the illness (Ch 11) is also important in organic cases.

DSM-IV does not include the term "organic brain syndromes" because it is thought to encourage a misleading separation between "organic" and "functional" states. DSM-IV uses the concept of "secondary" disorders instead.

CAUSES

- *Cerebral conditions*:
    - degenerative, for example senile and presenile dementias, Parkinson's disease
    - space-occupying lesions, for example primary brain tumour, cerebral metastases, subdural haematoma
    - infections, for example bacterial or viral meningitis or encephalitis, including HIV
    - head injury
    - epilepsy
    - vascular, for example arteriosclerosis, stroke, hypertensive encephalopathy, collagen diseases

- miscellaneous, for example multiple sclerosis, normal pressure hydrocephalus.
- *Systemic conditions*:
  - infections, for example septicaemia, pneumonia
  - metabolic disturbances, for example renal or hepatic failure, electrolyte imbalance, remote effects of carcinoma, porphyria
  - endocrine disorders, for example thyrotoxicosis, hypothyroidism, Cushing's syndrome
  - poisons, for example alcohol or drug intoxication or withdrawal, carbon monoxide, heavy metals
  - cardiac or respiratory conditions causing cerebral anoxia
  - vitamin B deficiency.

CLINICAL FEATURES

Organic cerebral disorders in which the whole brain is affected usually present with clouding of consciousness and/or cognitive impairment, which may be accompanied by neurological symptoms or signs. The classical picture in acute cases is called *delirium* and in chronic cases *dementia*. Localised lesions give rise to *focal impairments*. Delirium, dementia and focal syndromes are described below.

Less typical presentations include mood change, lability of mood, paranoid ideation, changes in behaviour or personality. Organic cases may present with neurotic or psychotic symptoms resembling those found in "functional" disorders, but often showing atypical features such as fluctuating symptomatology, visual hallucinations, vague or transient paranoid delusions, or first onset of neurotic symptoms in middle or old age. Cognitive testing may reveal unsuspected defects.

The symptom pattern depends more on the time course of the illness, and the part of the brain involved, than on the type of underlying pathology. Clinical features may also be modified by the patient's premorbid personality, premorbid vulnerability to psychiatric disorder, past life experience, current medication and social circumstances.

DELIRIUM

Definition

Delirium (acute brain syndrome, acute confusional state) is clouding of consciousness – that is, reduced awareness of the environment – accompanied by abnormalities of perception, thought and mood, from an organic cause. The alcohol withdrawal syndrome (delirium tremens) is a common example, but delirium may be due to any acute condition affecting the brain.

Clinical Features

The cardinal feature is a reduced level of consciousness. The patient is confused and disoriented, often restless, overactive and fearful but sometimes underactive and withdrawn. Inattention, including reduced ability to focus, sustain or shift attention, is common. Illusions, hallucinations of visual, auditory or tactile type, and changeable paranoid delusions may be present. Severity fluctuates, usually being worse at night.

Management

A first priority is diagnosis and treatment of the medical cause, for example diagnosing an occult infection, recognising withdrawal of alcohol or benzodiazepines, or identifying an adverse reaction to medication such as a tricyclic antidepressant or digitalis.

Nursing care, best carried out by one or two familiar people, is important. It includes attention to fluid intake and bladder and bowel function, provision of quiet warm well-lit surroundings without too many strange people around, protection against such hazards as unsupervised smoking in bed, and clear explanations before doing any practical procedures. Drug treatment, preferably with an antipsychotic started in low dose and increased as necessary, may be required to reduce disturbance or distress. Most cases are treated in general medical wards without involving psychiatrists.

Prognosis

Outcome depends on the cause and varies between complete recovery, partial recovery with residual dementia, and death. For general hospital inpatients, development of full-blown delirium is a predictor of increased mortality or, for those who survive, a prolonged hospital stay and/or need for subsequent placement in a nursing or residential home. Early detection and treatment of delirium is worthwhile.

DEMENTIA

Definition

Dementia (chronic brain syndrome) is an acquired global impairment of intellect and memory, often accompanied by changes in personality, mood and behaviour, from an organic cause. Dementia is usually progressive and irreversible, though some cases are due to treatable causes which are important to recognise.

Causes

The "primary dementias" include senile dementia of Alzheimer type, and the presenile dementias which include Alzheimer's disease, Pick's disease, Huntington's disease and the prion diseases. "Secondary dementia" may result from any of the conditions listed above as causing organic brain syndromes. The two most common types of dementia are Alzheimer's disease and vascular (multi-infarct, arteriosclerotic) dementia.

A general account of dementia is given below, followed by a description of some individual conditions.

Clinical Features

Onset is usually gradual, unless the dementia is the sequel of a delirious illness. Memory loss is usually the first symptom. This involves recent rather than remote memories, and results in disorientation.

Other intellectual functions also deteriorate. Affective changes are common, and may consist either of lability of mood, or a sustained depression or euphoria. Exaggeration of previous personality traits, and a coarsening of personality accompanied by socially unacceptable behaviour, may occur. Insight is usually absent, except in the early stages. Except in terminal cases, consciousness is unimpaired.

"Cortical" and "subcortical" types of dementia may be distinguished. Cortical dementia includes disturbance of "higher functions", for example dysphasia, agnosia and apraxia. In subcortical dementia these functions are preserved, but the patient is forgetful, slow and apathetic and may show marked emotional lability with sudden outbursts of laughter or rage.

Diagnosis

Diagnosis is made on clinical grounds from the history and mental state examination including simple cognitive testing. Formal psychometric tests can be used to confirm the diagnosis and specify the type of defects present, and repeated at intervals to monitor progress.

Investigation

All cases require a full medical history and physical examination. Treatable causes (such as brain tumour, subdural haematoma, normal pressure hydrocephalus, infections, hypothyroidism or vitamin B12 deficiency) may be revealed by investigations such as blood count and ESR, urea and electrolytes, liver function tests, thyroid function tests, B12 and folate, calcium and phosphate, serological tests for syphilis, HIV antibody testing (with informed consent), chest X-Ray, EEG and brain scan.

Potentially treatable lesions can be identified in about 10% of demented inpatients, but good results from treatment are obtained in about 2% only. Not all patients can be fully investigated for economic reasons; CT brain scans, routine in some other countries, are done selectively in the UK. Expensive or invasive investigations are only indicated if their results would alter management, and are seldom justified in patients whose dementia is very severe or whose general physical state is very poor.

Differential Diagnosis

Depression is the main condition liable to be confused with dementia, especially in the elderly. Depression and dementia can usually be distinguished by the history, mental state, and psychological testing, but in some patients the two disorders co-exist. In doubtful cases a therapeutic trial of antidepressant drugs or ECT should be undertaken.

Management

The cause of the dementia should be corrected if possible, but in the majority of cases no specific treatment exists. The aim of management is therefore to keep patients functioning at their optimum level by maintenance of good physical health and provision of a suitable environment. Availability of long-term inpatient care is limited, and in any case it is often best for patients to remain in their own homes with help from community services (Ch 20, Ch 26), as admission to hospital or nursing home may worsen their confusion and distress. The burden on relatives can be lessened by arranging short respite (holiday) admissions every few months, and offering prompt emergency admission in the event of an intercurrent illness or a social crisis.

Prognosis

In the minority of patients with a treatable cause, progression of the dementia can be arrested and there may even be partial recovery, but most cases gradually deteriorate. Acute confusional episodes due to other pathology, such as chest or urinary infections, strokes, faecal impaction, or inappropriate medication may be superimposed.

Specific types of dementia will now be described.

Senile Dementia of Alzheimer Type (SDAT)

Epidemiology: SDAT accounts for about half of all cases of dementia in old age. It is present in 5% of people over age 65 and 20% of people over 80. Women are affected nearly twice as often as men.

Cause: genetic predisposition exists and a link with allele e4 of apolipoprotein E on chromosome 19 has recently been reported. However, most cases are probably polygenic and multifactorial.

Neuropathology: shrinkage of the brain causes enlargement of the ventricles and sulci. Microscopically, there are three characteristic changes: neuronal loss, senile plaques and neurofibrillary tangles. Neurones are decreased both in number and size, and astrocytes proliferate. Senile plaques, which have argyrophilic cores containing an amyloid-like substance, develop in the grey matter. Nerve fibres form tangles called Alzheimer's neurofibrillary degeneration.

Oval structures called Lewy bodies are present in some cases and it is uncertain whether these represent a variant of SDAT or a variant of Parkinson's disease.

Neurochemistry and neurophysiology: postmortem brain studies show a deficiency of the enzyme choline acetyltransferase, which is concerned in the synthesis of acetylcholine, and defective cholinergic transmission is considered the likely basis of the symptoms.

Cerebral blood flow and oxygen consumption are reduced. The EEG usually shows theta or delta waves, with alpha rhythm slow or absent. Brain scan shows cerebral atrophy, selectively affecting the medial temporal lobe in early cases.

Symptoms: onset is gradual, over a year or more. Loss of recent memory is usually the first symptom, and is followed by deterioration in other mental functions, emotional lability or sustained depression, and personality change. Delusions and hallucinations, fits and neurological signs may occur in advanced cases. Insight is usually absent, and the patient comes to medical attention because relatives or neighbours notice failing memory, confusion, poor hygiene and self-neglect. Diagnosis is made on clinical grounds as there is no laboratory test for Alzheimer's disease, though tests may be required to exclude other causes of dementia.

In the Lewy body variant, Parkinsonian features are present; conscious level and cognitive function tend to fluctuate; and visual illusions or hallucinations may occur.

Treatment: many drugs, most of which enhance cholinergic activity, have been tried and the most promising, not yet licensed, is tacrine (tetrahydroaminoacridine, THA) which improves intellectual function in some cases but carries a risk of liver damage.

Prognosis: most patients die from pneumonia about five years after the onset of their dementia.

Presenile Alzheimer's Disease

Epidemiology: Alzheimer's disease is the commonest of the primary presenile dementias. Onset is between the ages of 40 and 60, and women are affected at least twice as often as men.

Causes: most cases arise sporadically but others are inherited, usually in polygenic fashion, in a few families by a dominant gene. Mutations in the amyloid precursor protein (APP) gene on chromosome 21 has been found in a few affected families and this is consistent with the observation that Trisomy 21 (Down's syndrome) (Ch 19) patients have an excess risk of developing Alzheimer's. In other families a gene on chromosome 14 appears responsible.

Neuropathology: the same as for senile Alzheimer's.

Clinical features: memory disturbance is the first symptom and develops gradually over two or three years. Rapid intellectual deterioration with symptoms of parietal lobe dysfunction (dysphasia, apraxia, agnosia, acalculia), accompanied by extrapyramidal signs, follows. Terminal cases have severe dementia and marked neurological abnormalities. The EEG is always abnormal, with theta and delta waves and reduced alpha rhythm.

Prognosis: death occurs within two to five years.

Vascular Dementia

Vascular dementia is almost as common as senile dementia, and the two conditions frequently co-exist.

Epidemiology: arteriosclerotic dementia usually starts between the ages of 60 and 70 but sometimes much earlier. Men are affected slightly more often than women.

Pathology: focal infarction of the brain due to haemorrhage, thrombosis or embolism, usually associated with cerebral arteriosclerosis. There may be a single CVA, or multiple small infarcts, or small vessel disease causing white matter damage. Most patients have hypertension, focal neurological signs, and evidence of arteriosclerosis in other organs.

Symptoms: loss of memory, intellectual deterioration and mood changes occur. Insight and personality are retained longer than for Alzheimer's disease, and the continued insight may contribute to the depression which is often present. Deterioration is stepwise rather than gradual, as repeated small strokes or episodes of hypertensive encephalopathy occur and leave residual damage.

Prevention and treatment: some cases might be prevented by control of hypertension in its early stages, and by attention to potential sources of emboli to the brain. Some improvement in the established condition may be achieved by treatment of very high blood pressure levels, cessation of smoking, and regular low-dose aspirin.

Prognosis: average survival time is about five years, and usual causes of death are ischaemic heart disease and stroke.

Pick's Disease

Pick's disease is a rare condition, probably caused by a dominant gene. Onset is between the ages of 50 and 60, and women are affected twice as often as men. Cerebral atrophy occurs, with loss of neurones and gliosis, most marked in the frontal and temporal lobes.

Symptoms of frontal lobe damage occur first and are followed by impairment of memory and intellect. Dysphasia, apraxia, agnosia and extrapyramidal symptoms are sometimes present. Death follows two to ten years after the onset.

Huntington's Disease (Huntington's Chorea)

Huntington's disease is a rare form of inherited presenile dementia. Its molecular genetics, and their clinical implications, have been extensively studied.

Epidemiology: 5 per 100 000 of the population are affected, with marked regional variation. Men and women are equally at risk.

Cause: an autosomal dominant gene with about 90% penetrance, located on the short arm of chromosome 4. The number of repeat sequences of the abnormal DNA triplicate (CAG) has some relationship to the age of onset, and severity, of the clinical disorder. Half the children of an affected parent will develop the condition, and because the age of onset is usually in mid-life, many patients have already had children themselves by the time symptoms begin. Occasionally patients have no family history, and such cases may be explained by spontaneous mutations or concealed illegitimacy.

Neuropathology and neurophysiology: generalised atrophy of the brain is most severe in the frontal lobes, caudate nuclei, and putamen. Low energy metabolism in the caudate nucleus, identified by PET scan, is characteristic and could be used as a presymptomatic test. Deficiency of GABA, and excess of dopamine, have been demonstrated at post-mortem.

Clinical features: onset may be at any age, but most often in mid-life (mean age 49). The juvenile form, starting in adolescence, accounts for 10% of cases. Choreiform movements and dementia are the most characteristic symptoms but there may be any type of psychiatric abnormality, for example neurotic, depressive or schizophrenic symptoms or psychopathic personality features, and great variation in the clinical course.

Treatment: choreiform movements can be modified with phenothiazines or tetrabenazine. Any psychiatric symptoms present should be treated with appropriate drugs.

Diagnosis: presymptomatic testing using genetic probes is now available through departments of medical genetics. The test may be carried out on an adult individual or an unborn child. Testing raises ethical issues, since there is no means of preventing or treating the disorder in those carrying the gene, and tests should only be carried out in the context of thorough family counselling. In practice, only a minority of at-risk individuals choose to be tested.

Prognosis: average survival time is about 15 years.

Prion Diseases: the Transmissible Dementias

Human examples of these disorders include *Creutzfeld–Jacob* (*Jacob–Creutzfeld*) disease, *kuru* (found in the cannibals of Papua New Guinea), *Gerstmann–Straussler–Scheinker* syndrome and *fatal familial insomnia*. Animal examples include *scrapie* in sheep, and *bovine spongiform encephalopathy* (BSE, "mad cow disease") described in British cattle in the 1980s and probably due to use of scrapie-infected sheep products in cattle-feed.

Causes: in some families, these dementias appear to be due to an inherited prion gene mutation which follows an autosomal dominant pattern. Other cases are infective, due to an abnormal prion protein acquired in various ways. The disorders can be transmitted to experimental animals, and a few human cases have developed following neurosurgery, corneal grafting, or administration of cadaveric growth hormone. Some authorities fear an imminent epidemic due to consumption of BSE-infected beef products.

Neuropathological features: prion protein, a modified cell membrane protein, accumulates within the CNS. There is neuronal loss, astrocytic hyperplasia and spongiform vacuolation in grey matter, with amyloid plaques.

Clinical features: dementia, accompanied by myoclonus or ataxia, usually starts in middle life. EEG changes are characteristic, and diagnosis can be confirmed by finding a prion gene mutation in a blood sample. These diseases are always fatal.

HIV Dementia

Cognitive impairment is very commonly associated with HIV infection and AIDS. About 10% of patients in the late stages of this illness develop a frank dementing syndrome due to invasion of the brain with the HIV virus. Typical features include forgetfulness, slowness and apathy, accompanied by motor weakness, with multiple neurological abnormalities in the later stages. Cerebral atrophy is shown on brain scan. Treatment with high-dose zidovudine (AZT) may bring about worthwhile clinical improvement. Differential diagnosis in the HIV-positive patient includes other cerebral infections such as toxoplasmosis, cryptococcus, cytomegalus or herpes simplex; cerebral lymphoma; also depressive illness. Specific treatments are available for several of these conditions, therefore it is desirable to reach an accurate diagnosis.

FOCAL BRAIN DAMAGE

Amnesic syndrome

The amnesic syndrome usually results from lesions of the posterior hypothalamus, less often from bilateral hippocampal lesions.

Causes:

- *Thiamine deficiency*, usually secondary to *alcoholism*, occasionally secondary to other causes of nutritional deficiency. *Korsakov's syndrome* is an alternative term for such cases.
- *Carbon monoxide* poisoning.
- *Vascular* lesions.
- The aftermath of *hypoxia* (such as may follow anaesthetic accidents, or attempted suicide by hanging) or *hypoglycaemia*.
- *Encephalitis*.

Clinical features: memory for recent events is grossly impaired, but immediate recall and long-term memory are both preserved, as are other intellectual functions. Many patients confabulate, that is they conceal their memory defect by elaborate falsifications.

Treatment: thiamine may be helpful if thiamine deficiency is present. Memory aids may enable some patients to function adequately but many need constant supervision.

Frontal Lobe Lesions

Personality change is often the first sign of a frontal lobe lesion. Behaviour becomes disinhibited, tactless or ill-judged; mood is inappropriately euphoric; drive and concentration are diminished, although there is no formal intellectual impairment; insight is lacking.

Neurological signs include a grasp reflex, anosmia, optic atrophy and incontinence. If the lesion involves the motor cortex there may be epileptic fits or contralateral spastic paresis.

Temporal Lobe Lesions

Personality change may take the form of increased aggression and emotional lability, or resemble that seen with frontal lobe lesions.

Temporal lobe epilepsy may develop. This condition, even more than other types of epilepsy, has important psychiatric aspects. It has an association with neurotic disorders, mood disorders, and schizophrenia, and a high suicide rate.

Intellectual deficits can be verbal or non-verbal depending which side is involved. Memory defects occur with bilateral lesions.

Neurological impairments include contralateral homonymous upper quadrant visual field defect, contralateral limb weakness or sensory loss, and language difficulties in the case of dominant hemisphere lesions.

Psychiatric symptoms of schizophrenic or affective type may occur.

FURTHER READING

Books

Burns A, Levy R (eds) (1993) *Dementia*. Chapman & Hall: London
Harper PS (ed) (1991) *Huntington's Disease*. WB Saunders: London
Lishman WA (1987) *Organic Psychiatry: Psychological Consequences of Cerebral Disorder* (2nd edn). Blackwell Scientific Publications: Oxford

Review Articles

Davison K (1989) Acute organic brain syndromes. *British Journal of Hospital Medicine* **41**: 89–92

Hardy JA, Davies DC (1988) Alzheimer's disease. *British Journal of Hospital Medicine* **39**: 372–377

Kopelman MD (1995) The Korsakoff syndrome. *British Journal of Psychiatry* **166**: 154–173

St Clair D (1994) Genetics of Alzheimer's disease. *British Journal of Psychiatry* **164**: 153–156

Whalley LJ (1989) Drug treatments of dementia. *British Journal of Psychiatry* **155**: 595–611

11

Psychiatric Aspects of Medical and Surgical Disease

Psychiatric disorders including anxiety, depression and/or organic brain syndromes are present in up to 50% of any population of medical or surgical patients. Some disorders are mild and transient but 10–20% of patients are severely affected. The majority of cases identified by research surveys are not receiving psychiatric treatment, and apparently have not been recognised by medical or nursing staff. This psychiatric "co-morbidity" adds to patients' suffering and, because it tends to be associated with a poor response to medical treatments and with extended hospital stays, it adds to healthcare costs.

The association between psychiatric and physical conditions may be explained in several ways:

- *Pre-existing psychiatric illness* or *personality disorder* may have played a role in causing the physical disorder, or hindering its recovery (see below).
- *The stress of the physical illness* (see below) may precipitate psychiatric disorder.
- *An organic brain syndrome* (Ch 10) has developed secondary to the physical illness or its treatment.
- *Somatic presentation* of a primary psychiatric condition (Ch 9), rather than a true medical or surgical diagnosis, is causing the symptoms.

The links between medical and psychiatric illness are reflected in the raised suicide rate of some, but not all, medical conditions: high-risk disorders include HIV/AIDS, cancers, especially of the head and neck, Huntington's disease, multiple sclerosis, peptic ulcer, renal failure, spinal cord injury and systemic lupus erythematosus (SLE). Primarily neurological conditions such as epilepsy are even more likely to be associated with psychiatric problems.

PSYCHOLOGICAL INFLUENCES ON THE COURSE OF PHYSICAL DISEASE

The question of whether psychological factors are directly linked to the development or prognosis of physical disease is controversial, and difficult to study. Classing certain illnesses as "psychosomatic" is no longer accepted, but psychological factors can certainly make an indirect contribution by their effects on lifestyle. Links include:

- *Behavioural factors*: patients with psychiatric illness or abnormal personalities are especially prone to:
    - voluntary behaviour which endangers health, such as heavy smoking and drinking, reckless driving
    - poor compliance with medical management of disease, for example delay in reporting new symptoms, failure to take tablets or follow lifestyle advice.

All psychiatric disorders carry a raised mortality, with about 80% of the excess being due to physical illness and about 20% to accidents or suicide.

- *Personality and attitudes*: some research studies suggest that "Type A" personalities (aggressive, impatient, competitive workaholics) have an increased risk of coronary heart disease; and that people who tend to repress their emotions, especially anger, have an increased risk of developing cancer. Other research suggests that patients with established cancer tend to live longer if they adopt a "fighting spirit" stance against their illness than if their response is a "helpless-hopeless" one. The validity of these associations remains disputed; there are difficulties in establishing the direction of cause and effect in studies of this kind, and behavioural factors such as degree of treatment compliance might account for any links which are found.

- *Life events*, and *social stress*: mortality and morbidity increase following major adverse life events such as bereavement. This may reflect changes in behaviour, such as self-neglect or deliberate self-harm, or might have a direct physiological basis, for example hormonal or immunological change.

THE STRESSES OF PHYSICAL ILLNESS

Any physical illness, and/or its treatment, can give rise to multiple losses and threats:

- *Unpleasant physical symptoms* such as pain, breathlessness or nausea.
- *Body-image problems*, for example weight loss or weight gain, surgical removal of a body part.
- *Biological influences on cognition and mood* due to brain disease, metabolic disturbance, or drugs such as steroids.
- *Enforced restrictions of lifestyle*, causing boredom or loss of self-esteem as well as practical and financial problems.
- *Interpersonal problems*, involving changed family dynamics and sexual relationships.
- *Concern and uncertainty* about future prognosis. Some patients are also troubled by existential and spiritual issues in relation to, for example, the reasons for their illness or the prospect of death and dying.
- *A sense of stigma*, attached most strongly nowadays to HIV/AIDS but also to many other physical disorders, for example epilepsy, skin disease.

ADJUSTMENT AND COPING

Many patients show emotional adjustment reactions following the first presentation of a physical illness, or its subsequent progression. Anxiety is common in the early stages, when symptoms have been noticed but no firm diagnosis made. If investigations confirm that a serious, progressive medical condition is present, some patients are actually relieved to know what they have to face. Others, not having suspected their diagnosis previously, go through a period of "denial" in which they do not seem to appreciate the gravity of the situation, and/or experience acute distress or anger. This is followed by depression or sadness before the final stage of acceptance can be reached. The pattern and the time course of the adjustment process varies

markedly, depending on many factors: the nature of the physical illness, the patient's personality and social circumstances, and relationships with healthcare staff.

The majority of patients with serious physical disease adjust successfully, through a variety of "coping styles". In general, those who
take positive action towards understanding and mastery of their illness tend to adapt better than those whose reaction is passive or
helpless. Sometimes the illness brings psychological benefits such as
closer family relationships, keener appreciation of life and a sense of
greater maturity. A minority of patients show persistent "maladaptive" reactions which may include anxiety, depression, anger or
denial. These always impair quality of life, and may cause poor
cooperation with, and response to, medical treatments.

Even patients who remain well after initial treatment for a serious
disease such as cancer may have their lives permanently overshad-
owed by fear of recurrence and death, and become hypochondriacal
about minor bodily symptoms. When incurable progressive disease
is a reality, many physical, psychological, social and spiritual issues
arise and the palliative care (hospice) movement is concerned with
optimising all these aspects of care for patients with advanced cancer
and other serious illnesses.

CLINICAL DEPRESSION IN MEDICALLY ILL PATIENTS

Depression is common but there are no agreed diagnostic criteria.
Two main difficulties arise:

- Distinguishing pathological mood disorder from appropriate
  sadness and adjustment.
- Determining the cause of somatic symptoms such as anorexia,
  loss of energy and sleep disturbance, which could be due to
  either mood disorder or the physical illness, or both.

If depressed mood is extremely severe, and/or prolonged more than
a few weeks after the patient receives bad news about his or her condition, depressive illness (clinical depression) should be suspected.
Detection of clinical depression is important because good relief of
symptoms can often be achieved with antidepressant drugs.

Key symptoms suggesting clinical depression in the physically ill
include guilt, perceiving the illness as a punishment, hopelessness,
loss of interest, loss of pleasure (anhedonia), inability to feel warmth

towards family and friends, or suicidal ideation. Depression sometimes presents with exacerbation of physical symptoms, for example difficult-to-control pain.

If a physically ill person requests euthanasia, or makes a suicide attempt, it is important to exclude clinical depression as well as making sure that the best possible medical and social care has been given.

MANAGEMENT AND PREVENTION

- *General approach*: patients often perceive deficiencies in their relationship and communication with healthcare professionals. Time to express concerns to a sympathetic listener, ask questions about the physical illness and its treatment and receive honest answers, may be all the treatment required for milder cases. Better provision of information to medical and surgical patients may help prevent psychiatric problems developing.
- *Recognising organic brain syndromes* (Ch 10): psychological disturbances secondary to biological factors may be reversible, but are often missed.
- *Psychological therapies* (Ch 22): cognitive-behavioural approaches are effective, and widely used. Brief psychodynamic therapy is indicated for a few with more complex or deep-seated problems.

Interventions have been used preventively, for enhancing psychological adjustment in the majority, and preventing psychiatric morbidity in the few. These include monitoring by nurse-counsellors, and supportive/educational group discussions for those with a particular physical condition, either with a professional therapist or on a self-help basis. There is some evidence that such measures reduce psychiatric symptoms, and improve "quality of life"; however not all patients want them.

- *Psychotropic drugs* (Ch 23): antidepressants are especially useful. Even for patients who have good cause to be depressed, these drugs can help improve mood, and relieve associated symptoms such as insomnia and pain. Antipsychotic drugs are used to control agitation or behaviour disturbance in patients with organic brain syndromes.
- *ECT* (Ch 24) is occasionally indicated for relief of severe depression, and is safe in physically ill patients provided they are fit for anaesthetic and do not have raised intracranial pressure.

LIAISON PSYCHIATRY

Liaison psychiatrists work with medical and surgical staff, and may have their own multidisciplinary teams of clinical psychologists, social workers and specialised psychiatric nurses. Their role includes:

● *Assessing and treating referred patients.* A recent report by the Royal College of Physicians and the Royal College of Psychiatrists classified clinical problems into the following groups:
  – organic disease with associated psychiatric disorder
  – cerebral complications of organic disease
  – bodily symptoms not due to organic disease (medically unexplained symptoms)
  – abuse of alcohol and drugs
  – deliberate self-harm (DSH)
  – sexual or relationship problems; eating disorders.

● *Educating general hospital staff* about recognising psychiatric disorder and the principles of its management.

● *Implementing screening programmes* for detection of psychiatric disorder, for example asking all patients to complete the Hospital Anxiety and Depression (HAD) Scale and interviewing the high scorers.

● *Research* into relationships between medical and psychiatric illness.

● *Staff support*: helping to address work-related problems and stress.

Space does not permit individual medical conditions to be considered here. Many psychiatric studies have been carried out, for example on HIV/AIDS, cancer, cardiac disease, diabetes, epilepsy, Parkinson's disease, renal failure, skin diseases, stroke; each condition has some unique features but similar general principles apply to them all.

FURTHER READING

Books

Lacey JH, Burns T (eds) (1989) *Psychological Management of the Physically Ill.* Churchill Livingstone: Edinburgh
Lloyd GG (1991) *Textbook of General Hospital Psychiatry.* Churchill Livingstone: Edinburgh

Royal College of Physicians and the Royal College of Psychiatrists (1995)
The Psychological Care of Medical Patients. Available from Royal College of Physicians Publications Unit, 11 St Andrews Place, London NW1 4LE

Review Articles

Harris EC, Barraclough BM (1994) Suicide as an outcome for medical disorders. *Medicine* **73**: 281–296

Mayou RA, Hawton K (1986) Psychiatric disorder in the general hospital. *British Journal of Psychiatry* **149**: 172–190

Rodin G, Voshart K (1986) Depression in the medically ill: an overview. *American Journal of Psychiatry* **143**: 696–705

12
Drug Misuse

DEFINITIONS

Drug misuse implies the use of drugs outside social, medical or legal norms. It is widespread among young people in the UK, and strongly linked with violent and criminal behaviour. Relevant terms include:

- *Addiction*: dependence on drugs with consequent detriment to social, physical or economic function.
- *Dependence*: psychological dependence is a strong desire to take a certain drug to produce pleasure or relieve distress, and physical dependence is indicated by the development of bodily symptoms if the drug is withdrawn.
- *Tolerance*: physical adaptation to a drug, leading to a need for increasing dosage to achieve the same effect. Tolerance often precedes development of physical dependence.

EPIDEMIOLOGY

- *Age*: illegal drug-taking is largely a problem of adolescents and young adults; up to 50% of teenagers experiment with illegal drugs but most have stopped using by their 20s. Although older people occasionally continue with illegal drugs, even up to their 50s or 60s, a much greater problem in middle and old age is the misuse of alcohol and of prescribed medication.

- *Sex*: illegal drug-taking is about four times more common in men. Misuse of prescribed drugs may be more common in women.

CAUSES

Psychological and social factors such as disordered personality, disturbed family background, membership of social groups in which drug-taking is prevalent, and ready availability of drugs whether through the black market or misguided medical prescribing, appear to be the main causes. A small minority of health professionals become addicted to narcotics and other substances (including anaesthetic gases, veterinary preparations) which they obtain at work.

PSYCHIATRIC AND PHYSICAL COMPLICATIONS

A history of drug misuse is often found nowadays in young male patients presenting with serious mental illnesses such as schizophrenia and schizo-affective disorders. Such patients may be especially prone to violent behaviour. In some, the drug misuse appears to have triggered the psychosis; others have used the drugs as self-medication for their psychotic symptoms.

Medical complications, sometimes fatal, often arise from the intravenous injections of opiates and other drugs. They include infections (abscesses, phlebitis, septicaemia, hepatitis, endocarditis, pneumonia and HIV), and arterial occlusions leading to gangrene of limbs. Drug misuse in pregnancy may be teratogenic, and lead to complications with the pregnancy or birth. Poor diet and poor hygiene in drug misusers lead to various impairments of health.

LEGAL ASPECTS

Chemicals with the potential for misuse can be classified according to their legal status:

- *Legal and freely available*: alcohol (Ch 13), tobacco, caffeine, solvents.
- *Sanctioned for medical use on prescription*: hypnotics, minor tranquillisers, opiates, anabolic steroids, anticholinergics especially procyclidine.

- *Illegal*, for example cannabis, cocaine.

The Misuse of Drugs Act 1971 governs the production, distribution, prescribing and possession of certain drugs. The drugs controlled under this Act are divided into Classes A, B and C, with Class A drugs being most dangerous and carrying the most severe penalties for misuse. The Act also distinguishes Schedules 1 through 5, which govern the rules for possession, storage, prescription and keeping of records. Further details are given in the *British National Formulary*.

The legal status of a drug may not be an accurate reflection of its dangerousness. Alcohol (Ch 13) and tobacco, which are legalised in this country and even socially encouraged in many settings, are possibly more threatening to life and health than some of the illegal substances considered in this chapter.

PHARMACOLOGY

Drugs which invite misuse fall into the following groups:

- *Opiates*.
- *Depressants and tranquillisers*, for example alcohol, barbiturates, chlormethiazole, benzodiazepines.
- *Stimulants*, for example cocaine, amphetamines, caffeine, khat.
- *Hallucinogens* (psychedelics, psychomimetics) for example LSD, mescaline, phencyclidine, psilocybin and psilocin (magic mushrooms).

Others include nicotine, cannabis, volatile inhalants, various "designer drugs". Many drug misusers take a mixture of drugs, the choice depending on availability, price and fashion as well as pharmacology.

PREVENTION

Much effort and expense have been devoted to educational presentations to schoolchildren, given by drug advisory bodies or specialised police officers; such programmes are designed to prevent drug misuse but could have the opposite effect on some individuals. They have not been demonstrated to be effective.

TREATMENT

While drug misuse can be seen as an illness requiring treatment, it is just as valid to regard it as a behaviour chosen by individuals, treatment for which will only succeed with the subject's motivation and cooperation. The Mental Health Act 1983 specifically excludes compulsory detention or treatment for drug addiction per se, though the Act does apply to mental disorders which have been caused by substance misuse.

The long-term aim of treatment may be either *complete abstinence* from drugs, or *controlled drug use*. Clients might be treated in dedicated inpatient settings, attend special outpatient clinics for controlled drug supplies, or consult community drug misuse teams staffed by specialised nurses and social workers with input from a consultant psychiatrist.

● *Abstinence*: if physical dependence is present, and the client elects to withdraw, initial treatment is often carried out in hospital. Withdrawal symptoms are avoided by stopping the drug gradually, and perhaps substituting another less harmful drug which has cross-tolerance with the original. Of psychological approaches to preventing relapse, most promising is the cognitive model which looks at situations and cues predisposing to resumption of drug use. A minority of addicts receive long-term treatment in residential units, which are run on therapeutic community lines and require members to abstain from drugs completely.

● *Controlled drug use*: many users do not wish to give up drugs, and the treatment aim is therefore "harm reduction". Advice would include instruction on safer injection techniques, giving out clean needles to reduce needle sharing, and encouraging change from injected to oral drugs. Some teams adopt an "assertive outreach" approach towards those drug users who lack the initiative to seek regular help for themselves.

Physical complications often need attention, and many addicts have social difficulties or personality problems for which extensive and prolonged help may be given, to uncertain effect. There are no accurate statistics on outcome of treatment, and results must be considered in relation to the natural history of drug misuse as a behaviour of adolescence and young adulthood which tends to die away in later life.

Individual drugs will now be described.

OPIATES

Opiates include morphine, heroin, methadone, pethidine, buprenor-
phine and dipipanone. Opium and morphine are derived from the
opium poppy, the others can be synthesised chemically.

Legal status and availability: strong opiates are Class A drugs but
some weaker ones are available over the counter as codeine preparations or in cough syrup. Most addicts obtain their supplies on the
black market but a few cases are iatrogenic due to inappropriate prescribing.

Administration: used to be mostly intravenous, but since awareness of
HIV, is more frequently by smoking or "snorting".

Psychological and social effects: intravenous injection may produce
either intense pleasure or malaise. Chronic opiate use leads to apathy, moodiness, and clouding of consciousness. Addicts' social circumstances deteriorate, and the need to obtain the drug dominates
their lives.

Physical effects: nausea, constipation, constricted pupils. Large doses
cause respiratory depression. Intravenous use may cause medical
complications as above. Use in pregnancy is associated with obstetric
complications: abrupt opiate withdrawal can cause intra-uterine
death, and opiate use at term causes respiratory depression and
withdrawal symptoms in the baby. Management of the pregnant
opiate user should include gradual withdrawal in the second
trimester if possible, with close cooperation between all the professionals concerned.

Tolerance and dependence: greatly increased tolerance, and physical
dependence, develop within a few weeks of starting regular use.
Endorphin neurotransmitters are probably involved. There is a
severe withdrawal syndrome consisting of craving, sleepiness, rhin-
orrhoea, lacrimation, abdominal colic and diarrhoea.

Detection: opiates can be detected by blood and urine tests.

Treatment: there is a legal requirement for all doctors to notify the
Home Office Drugs Branch, Queen Anne's Gate, London SW1H 9AT,

of opiate addicts with whom they come in contact. Maintenance prescriptions of *diamorphine* or *dipipanone* for addicts may only be issued by doctors with a special licence, working from a treatment centre, and it is advisable for the prescriptions to be dispensed from a designated pharmacy. (*Note*: any doctor may prescribe diamorphine for relief of severe pain.) *Methadone*, which is taken orally and may be prescribed by any doctor, is an alternative drug for maintenance. For those who continue to inject, many centres provide sterile needles free of charge under the "harm reduction" policies designed to restrict spread of HIV. For those who elect to withdraw, hospital admission is recommended, and *clonidine* or *lofexidine* may be given to control withdrawal symptoms. *Naltrexone*, an opioid antagonist, blocks the euphoriant effects of opioids and may therefore be taken on a long term basis as an aid to relapse prevention.

Prognosis: some opiate addicts give up their habit either spontaneously or with medical help. Mortality is increased about 15 times, the most frequent causes of death being respiratory depression from drug overdose, infections, and suicide.

AMPHETAMINES (SPEED)

Legal status and availability: injectable amphetamines are Class A, and oral amphetamines Class B drugs. They used to be widely prescribed for depression and obesity. There is now a voluntary ban on prescription, however private prescription by "slimming clinics" and easy chemical synthesis are responsible for continued widespread availability.

Administration: oral, intravenous or inhaled.

Psychological effects: amphetamines are stimulants which cause euphoria, increased activity, insomnia and anorexia. *Amphetamine psychosis* consists of visual or auditory hallucinations with paranoid delusions, similar to paranoid schizophrenia. (As amphetamines act by stimulation of CNS dopamine systems, this effect is a main plank of the "dopamine hypothesis" of schizophrenia.) Amphetamine psychosis nearly always recovers within a week if the drug is withdrawn.

Physical effects: stimulation of sympathetic nervous system activity.

Tolerance and dependence: psychological dependence and tolerance occur but probably not physical dependence. Depressed mood, low energy and increased sleep may follow withdrawal.

Detection: amphetamines can be detected by blood and urine tests.

COCAINE ("SNOW") AND CRACK

Cocaine is derived from the coca shrub grown in South America. Crack is cocaine which has been separated from its hydrochloride salt.

Legal status and availability: cocaine is a Class A drug, not used in medical practice except in ENT and related surgery.

Administration: inhaled as snuff or injected. Crack can be smoked to produce a rapid effect.

Psychological effects: similar to those of amphetamine. *Cocaine psychosis* resembles the amphetamine psychosis but also includes tactile hallucinations consisting of a sensation of insects crawling on the skin (formication).

Physical effects: cocaine may cause cardiac arrhythmias. Repeated inhalation may cause perforation of the nasal septum.

Tolerance and dependence: only psychological dependence occurs with ordinary cocaine, but crack is highly addictive and both tolerance and physical dependence rapidly develop.

Detection: cocaine can be detected by blood and urine tests.

Treatment: addicts should be notified to the Home Office. Maintenance prescriptions can only be issued by doctors with a special licence.

CANNABIS (INDIAN HEMP, HASHISH, POT)

Cannabis is the name given to products of the plant *Cannabis sativa*, which include hashish and marijuana. "Skunkweed" is an especially potent form. The psychoactive ingredient is *tetrahydrocannabinol* (THC). *Cannabis sativa* grows wild in many countries including Britain. THC can also be chemically synthesised.

Legal status and availability: cannabis is a Class B drug, but freely available from unofficial sources and probably used by at least 10% of young people in this country. Legalising cannabis is often suggested, because some experts do not believe it has serious adverse effects.

Administration: cannabis is usually mixed with tobacco and smoked, but can also be taken orally or intravenously.

Psychological and social effects: cannabis usually produces well-being, relaxation and sociability, but can exaggerate an unpleasant pre-existing mood state of anger, depression or anxiety. Perceptual distortions, visual hallucinations and confusion can occur. The use of cannabis is often implicated in worsening the clinical course of schizophrenia, precipitating onset or relapse and retarding recovery. Sustained long-term use is believed to cause an "amotivational syndrome" of apathy and cognitive defects, probably reversible if the drug is stopped.

Physical effects: cannabis has many physiological effects, including cardiovascular ones which may be dangerous in people with heart disease. Cannabis taken in pregnancy is thought to be teratogenic. Chronic effects include those of the associated tobacco smoking. Cannabis has antiemetic, anticonvulsant and analgesic properties which might well be useful in medical practice if doctors were allowed to prescribe.

Tolerance and dependence: psychological dependence is common. A withdrawal syndrome can occur after stopping long-term use.

Detection: cannabis can be detected in body fluids for up to two weeks after consumption.

Prognosis: occasional cannabis use appears harmless in most people, despite the concerns about psychotic illness described above. There is no evidence that cannabis predisposes directly to use of more dangerous drugs, however it may do so indirectly through encouraging contact with other drug users.

LYSERGIC ACID DIETHYLAMIDE (LSD, ACID)

LSD is a synthetic compound.

Legal status and availability: LSD is a Class A drug, no longer used in medical practice, but easily synthesised by amateur chemists.

Administration: oral.

Psychological effects: perceptual distortion, abreaction of distant memories, extreme depression or ecstasy ("bad trips" or "good trips"), acute psychotic experiences. Death can result, for example from delusions of being able to fly from high places. "Flashbacks" of LSD-induced experiences may continue for years after the last dose.

Physical effects: those of sympathetic nervous system overactivity.

Detection: LSD cannot be detected by laboratory tests.

Tolerance and dependence: do not occur.

MDMA (ECSTASY)

MDMA (3,4, methylenedioxyamphetamine) is a Class A "designer drug" which alters perceptual and emotional experience, giving enhanced appreciation of colour and sound and increased empathy with others, and also has stimulant properties. It is popular for use at pop festivals and "rave" parties, but may cause sudden death in such settings through cardiac arrhythmia, dehydration and hyperthermia. It may precipitate or cause psychosis. Long-term use may have neurotoxic effects. Dependence may develop.

GLUES AND SOLVENTS

Fumes from products based on toluene and acetone have been increasingly used for their psychological effects in recent years. Such products include glues and solvents for domestic or industrial use. They are freely available and popular among children, particularly male adolescents.

Administration: inhalation from paper, bottle or bag (glue-sniffing).

Psychological effects: euphoria and perceptual disturbance, progressing to stupor. Long-term neuropsychological damage may occur.

Physical effects: these substances are toxic to the liver, kidney, heart and brain, and inhalation may cause accidental death. Chronic use causes an acneiform rash around the mouth and nose.

Tolerance and dependence: psychological dependence is common, but tolerance and physical dependence probably do not occur.

TOBACCO

Nicotine is the constituent of tobacco which causes psychological effects and dependence, whereas carbon monoxide and tar cause the physical ill-effects. Cigarette smoking is more harmful than other forms of tobacco consumption. About one-third of the population smoke and rates are rising among young women. Smoking is widespread among patients and nurses in psychiatric hospitals.

Psychological effects: nicotine is both a central nervous system stimulant and an anxiolytic.

Physical effects: acute effects are those of sympathetic nervous system overactivity. Chronic effects include raised susceptibility to lung cancer and many other cancers, cardiovascular disease, chronic bronchitis and, during pregnancy, stillbirth and abortion.

Tolerance and dependence: both psychological and physical dependence occur. There is a withdrawal syndrome consisting of anxiety, depression, irritability, insomnia and craving.

Management: nicotine chewing-gum is a less toxic alternative which helps some smokers give up. Psychological methods including hypnosis and group therapy are sometimes effective. It would be better to prevent people from ever starting to smoke, through education in schools, banning advertisements, and increasing the price of cigarettes.

CAFFEINE

Caffeine, a xanthine alkaloid, is a constituent of coffee, tea, cocoa, and cola beverages. Most people in the UK consume several such drinks a day without apparent ill-effects.

Psychological effects: caffeine is a stimulant which increases well-being and reduces fatigue. Large doses cause anxiety and insomnia. "Caffeinism" is an important differential diagnosis of anxiety disorders. Some psychiatric patients consume large amounts (say 10 or 20 cups of tea or coffee daily) in the mistaken belief that this helps to calm their nerves.

Physical effects: tachycardia, diuresis, muscle tension.

Tolerance and dependence: psychological but not physical dependence occurs.

BARBITURATES

Legal status and availability: barbiturates used to be widely prescribed as tranquillisers and hypnotics before their addictive potential became clear. Their prescription for this purpose is now discouraged, though a few older people remain dependent. Barbiturates are still sometimes used for epilepsy. Black market barbiturates are less frequently used today.

Administration: oral or intravenous.

Psychological effects: central nervous system (CNS) depression causing psychomotor impairment, drowsiness or sleep.

Physical effects: ataxia, nystagmus, slurred speech. Large doses may cause fatal respiratory depression. Cross-tolerance with alcohol and anaesthetics exists.

Tolerance and dependence: tolerance and physical dependence develop rapidly. There is a withdrawal syndrome of anxiety, insomnia, tremor, fits and delirium.

Detection: barbiturates can be detected by blood and urine tests.

BENZODIAZEPINES

Misuse is currently an important problem: see Ch 23.

FURTHER READING

Books

Chick J, Cantwell R (1994) *Seminars in Alcohol & Drug Misuse*. Gaskell: London

Ghodse H (1989) *Drugs and Addictive Behaviour: a Guide to Treatment*. Blackwell Scientific Publications: Oxford

HMSO (1991) *Drug Misuse & Dependence: Guidelines & Clinical Management*. HMSO: London

Review Articles

Henry JA (1992) Ecstasy and the dance of death. *British Medical Journal* **305**: 5–6

Poole R, Brabbins C (1996) Drug induced psychosis. *British Journal of Psychiatry* **168**: 135–138

Ron MA (1986) Volatile substance abuse: a review of possible long-term neurological, intellectual and psychiatric sequelae. *British Journal of Psychiatry* **148**: 235–246

Strang J, Johns A, Caan W (1993) Cocaine in the UK. *British Journal of Psychiatry* **162**: 1–13

Thomas H (1993) Psychiatric symptoms in cannabis users. *British Journal of Psychiatry* **163**: 141–149

13
Alcohol Misuse

A moderate alcohol intake is, for most people, acceptable and enjoyable. Those who drink to excess, or are particularly vulnerable to the unwanted effects of alcohol, may experience a wide range of medical and psychiatric problems.

Alcohol misuse may be defined in terms of:

- *Quantity* of alcohol intake.
- Presence of *dependency*.
- Alcohol-related *disability*, whether physical, mental or social.

There is no agreed definition of "alcoholism", nor clear distinction between this and heavy drinking.

SAFE LIMITS OF DRINKING

Quantities: the limits of 21 units per week for men and 14 for women suggested by the Royal College of Physicians have been widely influential. A "unit" is one drink (half a pint of ordinary strength beer, one glass of wine or sherry, a single measure of spirits) and contains 8–10 g alcohol. Higher limits (28 for men, 21 for women) were recently suggested by the government, against advice from the medical profession.

Pattern: "binge drinking" can cause problems (for example accidents, especially head injury, acute alcoholic poisoning, and involvement in criminal activity such as assault and vandalism) over and above those found with the steady daily intake of equivalent amounts of alcohol.

FREQUENCY

Up to 5% of people in England and Wales have a serious drinking problem. About 25% of men and 15% of women drink more than the recommended limits given above.

Alcohol misuse is often concealed. Its extent within a given population can be estimated by:

- *Alcohol sales* per capita.
- Alcohol-related *hospital admissions*.
- *Drunkenness* convictions.
- Mortality from *cirrhosis of the liver*.

EPIDEMIOLOGY

- *Nationality*: wine-producing countries like France and Italy have high rates of alcohol-related problems. Muslim and Jewish societies, with their religious constraints on drinking, have low ones. Scotland and Ireland have higher rates than England and Wales.
- *Occupation*: groups at high risk include publicans, seamen, journalists and doctors.
- *Age*: most cases present in middle age, but a growing number of young adults are seeking treatment, and concealed alcohol misuse is increasingly recognised as a problem in old age.
- *Sex*: men are more often affected than women but the prevalence among women is increasing.

CAUSES

- *Genetics*: there is a 2–3-fold increase in alcoholism in the relatives of alcoholics, especially male ones; a higher concordance between monozygotic than dizygotic twins; and a high rate in children of alcoholic parents who were adopted into non-alcoholic homes in infancy. Sociopathic personality disorder is over-represented among the male relatives of alcoholics, and depressive illness among female relatives.

- *Psychological factors*: psychosocial stress is often the precipitant for heavy drinking, alcohol being a powerful temporary anxiolytic and euphoriant. Any psychiatric disorder may lead to self-medication with alcohol.
- *Social and cultural factors*: drinking problems are more common in settings where alcohol is cheap and easily available, and drinking is encouraged socially.
- *Economic*: the greater the per capita consumption of alcohol in a society, the larger is the number of people with alcohol problems, and per capita consumption is inversely related to price. This means that a nation's alcohol taxation policy affects its rate of alcohol-related problems.

EFFECTS OF ALCOHOL

Small quantities promote sociability and well-being, and may bring certain health benefits; people who take one or two drinks per day suffer less coronary heart disease and have a lower all-cause mortality rate than non-drinkers. Higher consumption, whether on a long-term regular basis or in the form of acute drunkenness, can cause many damaging effects.

Damage may result from direct toxicity of ethanol, or from associated phenomena including vitamin B deficiency, hypoglycaemia, dehydration, alcohol withdrawal, toxic congeners (other substances present in alcoholic drinks) and trauma sustained during intoxication.

Acute Intoxication

Blood alcohol levels around 50 mg% cause increased well-being, reduced inhibitions and reduced efficiency (seldom recognised by the subject).

Heavier intoxication causes obvious cognitive impairment, ataxia, slurred speech and vomiting, with subsequent amnesia.

Coma usually supervenes when blood alcohol reaches about 300 mg%. Coma in heavy drinkers may also result from head injury, drug overdose, a recent fit, hypothermia or hypoglycaemia.

Blood alcohol levels over 500 mg% may be fatal. Milder degrees of intoxication can lead to death indirectly through accidents or inhalation of vomit.

"Pathological intoxication" is abnormal behaviour following only modest alcohol intake, usually described in brain-damaged people, though there is doubt as to the validity of this concept.

Neuropsychiatric Complications

- *Delirium tremens* (DTs), an indication of physical dependence, can be precipitated by abrupt withdrawal of alcohol in a heavy drinker, for example the end of a drinking bout, efforts to give up drinking without professional advice, intercurrent illness, hospital admission, or arrest/imprisonment. Confusion, fever, visual or tactile hallucinations and fits may occur. Delirium tremens is a medical emergency with an appreciable mortality, and should be treated by physicians. Treatment includes correction of any fluid or electrolyte imbalance or hypoglycaemia, and a five-day reducing course of a benzodiazepine, such as chlordiazepoxide, to counteract withdrawal symptoms by sedation and prevention of fits. These drugs have potential for dependence and abuse, and should not be continued after detoxification. Parenteral vitamins, thiamine being most important, are also given to try to prevent other neurological complications.
- *Wernicke's encephalopathy* is an acute syndrome thought to result from deficiency of B1 (thiamine). Haemorrhages occur in the mammillary bodies, thalamus and hypothalamus. Acute confusion is accompanied by nystagmus, diplopia, ataxia and peripheral neuritis. The condition may be fatal unless promptly treated with thiamine.
- *Korsakov's syndrome*, a more chronic disorder, is also believed to result from thiamine deficiency. It may be a sequel of delirium tremens or Wernicke's encephalopathy. Haemorrhage, necrosis and gliosis are present in the mammillary bodies and hippocampus. A gross defect of short-term memory leads to disorientation, for which some patients attempt to compensate by confabulation. Peripheral neuropathy often co-exists.
- *Alcoholic dementia* comprises global impairment of mental functioning, often accompanied by personality changes of the frontal lobe type. Brain scan shows cerebral atrophy, partly reversible if the subject stops drinking.
- *Epilepsy* may be caused by direct toxicity of alcohol, especially if there is pre-existing brain damage; alcohol withdrawal; overhydration; or hypoglycaemia.

- *Peripheral neuropathy* results from thiamine deficiency, and affects motor, sensory and autonomic nerves. Presenting symptoms include impotence, or burning pain in the feet.

Other neurological complications include cerebellar degeneration, central pontine myelinosis, degeneration of the corpus callosum, retrobulbar neuritis, and subdural haematoma following falls.

- *Alcoholic hallucinosis* often starts during a phase of abstinence and recovers spontaneously after a few months. Auditory hallucinations, usually voices, develop in clear consciousness. If insight is lacking, the voices may form a basis for a delusional system.
- *Alcoholic paranoia* is the development of paranoid delusions in the absence of hallucinations. Morbid jealousy (Ch 8) of the sexual partner is a frequent theme, in which case dangerousness (Ch 21) must be assessed because of the risk of assault or even homicide.

Alcoholic hallucinosis and alcoholic paranoia can be controlled by antipsychotic drugs.

Physical Complications

The mortality rate in alcoholics is about three times the general population rate.

- *Liver damage* includes acute hepatitis, fatty infiltration, and cirrhosis. In men, cirrhosis seldom develops until heavy drinking has continued for at least five years, but women are more vulnerable. Cirrhosis has a high mortality rate even in those who become totally abstinent.
- *In pregnancy,* heavy drinking may cause abortion, stillbirth, or the "foetal alcohol syndrome" comprising microcephaly and other deformities, and learning disability.

Other physical consequences include peptic ulcer, pancreatitis, gastritis, cardiomyopathy, myopathy, gout, vitamin deficiencies, drug interactions (the effect of psychotropic drugs may be either enhanced or reduced) and raised susceptibility to infections, including tuberculosis, and malignancies.

Accidents, including road accidents, and *accidental deaths* are common. *Suicide* is the cause of death in about 15% of alcoholics, and 50% of non-fatal self-poisonings are combined with alcohol.

Social Consequences

- *Family disruption*: marital breakdown, and violence towards partners and children.
- *Working efficiency* is reduced, often leading to demotion or unemployment.
- *Crime*: many alcoholics steal to get money for drink, and intoxication may precipitate violence. About 50% of violent crimes are committed when the offender is drunk, and about 50% of men in prison have a drinking problem.
- *Drunken driving*: 80 mg% is the legal upper limit of blood alcohol for drivers in the UK, which may be too lenient as driving skills are demonstrably impaired at 30 mg%.

COURSE OF ALCOHOL ABUSE

The traditional view, which may well apply to some of the most severely affected, is of a relentlessly progressive disorder. Alcohol problems commonly begin when social drinking becomes heavier for psychological reasons, such as living in a hard-drinking environment, or stressful work or family circumstances. This stage of psychological dependence is followed in some cases by development of physical dependence, manifest by loss of control over the amount consumed, and withdrawal symptoms (tremor, sweating, anxiety, craving) if alcohol is unavailable for a few hours. Intake increases further to combat withdrawal symptoms. Alcohol tolerance increases initially, decreasing again when the condition becomes advanced. Drinking gains priority over other activities, and the various physical, psychiatric and social problems ensue.

Other patterns include repeated relapses and remissions according to current circumstances and/or changes in mood. As with other kinds of substance misuse (Ch 12), some people drink heavily in early adulthood but "grow out" of their habit later on.

Many drinkers deny their problem, concealing the extent of their drinking and hiding bottles at home or at work.

Heavy smoking, dependence on other drugs, and heavy gambling may be associated.

Vagrant (skid row) alcoholics are those without families, homes, money or jobs, often handicapped by low intelligence or chronic mental illness, who live rough in city centres drinking cheap forms of alcohol.

RECOGNITION

Patients with undetected drinking problems commonly present in primary care or hospital settings because of the physical or psychiatric complications of alcohol. Patients with, for example, depressive illness or peptic ulcer will not improve if treatment is directed to these diagnoses without attention to the underlying alcohol misuse. Ways of improving recognition include:

- *Taking a drinking history* as a routine part of medical or nursing assessment.
- *Screening questionnaires* such as *CAGE*:

   Have you ever felt you ought to **C**ut down on your drinking?
   Have people **A**nnoyed you by criticising your drinking?
   Have you ever felt **G**uilty about your drinking?
   Have you ever had a drink first thing in the morning (an "**E**ye-opener") to steady your nerves or get rid of a hangover?

Two or more positive replies indicate a possible drinking problem, but must be followed up by direct inquiry. Brief counselling by trained nurses is effective in persuading general medical patients identified in this way to reduce their drinking.

- *Laboratory tests*: a raised blood level of the enzyme gamma glu-tamyltranspeptidase (gamma GT) (over 40 iu/litre), and/or macro-cytosis (mean corpuscular volume, MCV, over 96 fl), are suggestive of high alcohol intake, though both tests may also give abnormal results in certain medical illnesses unrelated to alcohol.

TREATMENT

Alcohol misuse cannot be regarded as a disease to be "cured" by doctors. The responsibility for change in behaviour rests with the drinker, the professional's role being to facilitate this change. There is little point in treating those who deny their problem, or do not want to overcome it. Some who are well motivated stop drinking of their own accord, others need professional help, but the strength of motivation is the most powerful predictor of treatment success.

Intervention is probably most effective at an early stage, but most alcohol misusers do not seek help till they are forced to do so and their condition is advanced. Once heavy drinking has become established and physical dependence is present, results of treatment are poor.

Total abstinence is the traditional goal, especially for those with physical dependence or physical complications. Controlled drinking is a realistic aim for some milder cases. Treatment methods include:

- *Detoxification*, using medical treatment as outlined above for delirium tremens, is necessary to permit safe cessation of drinking in those who are chemically dependent (as evidenced by a physical withdrawal syndrome). It may be done safely at home or in a hostel if there is adequate supervision. A typical regime would be chlordiazepoxide 60 mg qds, reducing gradually to zero over five days. Chlormethiazole (Hemineverin) was formerly the standard treatment, but is no longer recommended.

- *Psychological and social approaches*: systematic reviews indicate that most brief approaches are effective in reducing consumption, but that longer-term psychological treatments (including dynamic, behavioural or supportive psychotherapy, individual or group, on an inpatient or outpatient basis) have no additional benefit. The trend is firmly toward inexpensive community treatments with input from health, social and probation services. However, inpatient alcoholic units still exist, offering intensive group psychotherapy over several weeks or months. Long-term residence in a "dry" hostel offers support for some severely damaged ex-drinkers.

Alcoholics Anonymous (AA) is a voluntary organisation which offers self-help group therapy at evening meetings and also runs groups for partners and children. The goal of lifetime total abstinence is central to AA's approach. Some people derive great benefit from AA, and continue frequent attendance at meetings for many years to make sure they remain "dry". For others, however, the AA approach makes them feel so guilty if they return to drinking that they are more likely to continue doing so.

Motivational interviewing uses a model which can also be applied to other addictive behaviours, describing a "cycle of change":
- precontemplation
- contemplation
- action
- maintenance/relapse.

Problem drinking is seen as being likely to recur several times before the drinker gains control; returns to drinking are seen not as sinful but as learning experiences. This has the advantage of recognising that multiple attempts are often necessary before a drink problem can be mastered.

- *Drugs*: *disulfiram* ("Antabuse" tablets or implant) blocks the action of acetaldehyde dehydrogenase, causing accumulation of acetaldehyde if alcohol is taken. Drinking therefore becomes both unpleasant and dangerous, with the risk of cardiac arrhythmias or extreme hypotension. Disulfiram should only be prescribed to well-motivated patients who appreciate the risks of combination with alcohol; these may well have a good prognosis anyway. Other drugs which have been tried include *lithium* and *fluoxetine* and, more recently, *naltrexone* which detracts from the pleasurable effects of drinking. It has not yet been established that any of these drugs improve long-term outcome.

PROGNOSIS

Following treatment in an alcoholic unit with subsequent outpatient group support, about 30% of patients remain abstinent and another 30% are improved. Such patients have often been preselected as likely to benefit from intensive treatment and therefore represent a good-prognosis group. Poor prognostic features are female sex, youth, premorbid personality disorder and social isolation.

PREVENTION

There is evidence that a reduction in national per capita alcohol consumption, and hence a reduction in the number of people with alcohol-related problems, could be achieved by *increasing the price of alcohol*.

Other measures which may be presumed to be helpful include: *education* about the dangers of alcohol, *offering non-alcoholic drinks* at business and social functions, *banning advertisements* for drink, *tougher drink-drive laws*, and placing moderate (but not extreme) *restrictions on availability* in shops and catering establishments.

FURTHER READING

Chick J, Cantwell R (1994) *Seminars in Alcohol & Drug Misuse.* Gaskell: London

14

Deliberate Self-harm

Fatal deliberate self-harm (*suicide, completed suicide*) and *non-fatal* deliberate self-harm (*DSH, parasuicide, attempted suicide*) are separate phenomena which overlap to some degree. Both medical and social factors are involved in their aetiology, prevention and management.

SUICIDE

Definition

Suicide is an act of self-harm, undertaken with conscious self-destructive intent, with a fatal outcome.

Frequency

There are between 4000 and 5000 suicides in England and Wales per year; about 10 per 100 000 population, and 1% of all deaths. Official statistics underestimate the rate because only cases with proven evidence of intent, such as a suicide note, are given suicide verdicts by the coroner. Many deaths given "accident" or "undetermined" verdicts are probably suicides too.

Methods

Hanging/strangling/suffocation and gassing by car exhaust fumes (carbon monoxide), are now the most common methods taken over-all, although poisoning (often by medicinal drugs) remains the commonest method in women. Other methods include drowning, shooting, cutting, jumping and burning. Methods which are most easily available are most likely to be used, and media publicity about a suicide is often followed by other deaths using the same method.

Epidemiology

- *Age*: the rate increases with age, but suicide in young men (age 15–24) has recently become much more frequent.
- *Sex*: more than twice as common in men.
- *Marital status*: divorced people have the highest rates, followed by the widowed and single, and married the lowest.
- *Social class*: highest rates at both extremes of the social scale.
- *Occupation*: high-risk groups include doctors, vets, pharmacists and farmers.
- *Residential circumstances*: inner city areas with a mobile population have high rates. Inmates of psychiatric hospitals, patients recently discharged from such hospitals, and prisoners are all at high risk.
- *Nationality*: there are large differences between the suicide rates of different countries. These are partly real, due for example to religious and cultural variation, but some apparent differences result from differing methods of ascertainment. High rates are found in Greenland, Hungary, Austria, Denmark, Japan, Germany and Eastern Europe. Low rates are found in Eire, Italy, Spain, Greece and the Netherlands.
- *National circumstances*: suicide rates fall in wartime. High suicide rates are found in association with economic depression, unemployment, and high divorce rates.
- *Season*: highest rates in springtime.

Causes

- *Psychiatric disorder*: present immediately before death in up to 90% of cases, as indicated by the "psychological autopsy" technique of interviewing those who knew the dead person. Depressive illness, often inadequately treated, is the commonest diagnosis, especially in older people. Alcohol and drug misuse are also common, especially in the young. Personality disorder often co-exists. "Rational" suicide, by mentally normal people in hopeless situations, is rare in Western societies but more often found in Oriental ones.

Follow-up of psychiatric patient populations indicates that in 5–15% of subjects with mental illness, personality disorder and/or drug or alcohol problems, suicide will be the cause of death.

● *Stressful circumstances*, including life events such as bereavement, and long-term social difficulties such as unemployment.

● *Social isolation*, in those who live alone and/or lack confiding relationships.

● *Physical illness*: raised suicide rates are found in association with certain physical conditions, including epilepsy, other neurological disorders, peptic ulcer, renal failure on dialysis, and AIDS.

● *Neurochemistry*: deficiency of 5-HT has been linked to suicidal behaviour in some studies.

The French sociologist Emile Durkheim, whose influential book *Le Suicide* was published in 1894, distinguished three types: "anomic" related to a disorganised society, "egoistic" among people isolated from their social group, and "altruistic" for the benefit of others.

More recent research suggests that the psychological state of *hopelessness* is a key precursor of suicide.

Prevention

Some preventive strategies aim to improve the management of individuals at high risk, others to reduce factors associated with suicidality in society as a whole. Reduction of suicide rates, both for the general population and for psychiatric patients, is among the targets in the government's "Health of the Nation" strategy.

● *Medical care of the mentally ill*: many suicides have been in contact with GPs or psychiatrists shortly before death, raising the possibility that better medical management might have prevented the fatal act. Psychiatric patients who have voiced suicidal thoughts, have a past history of suicide attempts, or possess the sociodemographic factors listed above should be considered at high risk.

Prompt and energetic physical treatment of psychiatric illness should help prevent suicide in the mentally ill. High doses of psychotropic drugs may be required, but potentially suicidal patients should not be given large supplies which might be used in overdose. ECT may be indicated for the suicidally depressed. In the long term, lithium prophylaxis helps to reduce the suicide risk for people prone to recurrent depression

Suicidal patients who live with responsible relatives or friends can often be managed at home, but must have frequent follow-up reviews, and 24-hour access to professional help in case of emergency. Hospital admission, with close nursing observation, is indicated for the very severely ill and those without adequate home support.

In cases where more chronic psychiatric and social problems existed, a growing alienation from professional carers sometimes seems to have been a factor in the suicide. This can happen if staff themselves become hopeless or cynical in relation to an unrewarding case, and points to the importance of ongoing supportive care in suicide prevention.

- *Counselling services*, such as the confidential telephone helplines for despairing and suicidal people run by the Samaritan organisation.
- *Restricting availability of methods*, such as catalytic converters for cars; controls on sales and possession of medicines, guns and poisons; designing hospitals so that psychiatric wards are at ground-floor level; preventing public access to bridges or clifftops from which others have jumped to their deaths. Removal of a method can have a significant long-term effect as it is not necessarily replaced by other methods; during the 1960s, changing the domestic gas supply from coal gas (containing carbon monoxide) to non-toxic natural gas was followed by a sustained reduction in total UK suicide rate.
- *Restricting media reports* about suicide.
- *Educational programmes*, for example to improve the recognition and management of potentially suicidal patients in general practice, or to dissuade young people from suicidal behaviour.

Individual preventive strategies are difficult to evaluate because so many factors affect the suicide rate.

The Aftermath of Suicide

Bereavement counselling and practical help may be required in the immediate aftermath of the death, which will almost always be a very difficult time for relatives. In the longer term, the relatives of those who died by suicide are at high risk of psychiatric illness and social problems and many take years to adjust, if ever they do, to a death which frequently seems like an act of aggression as well as of self-destruction. Others however ultimately find their lives made easier, for example if the dead person had been affected for many years by a severe and intractable personality disorder, mental illness or drug/alcohol misuse.

The professionals involved often react with distress and guilt, understandable but not always justified. A certain number of suicides are bound to occur in psychiatric practice, and it is not possible to predict exactly which individuals are going to kill themselves, or when. After a suicide has taken place, review of the case may well suggest some way that management could have been improved; this should be used as a constructive opportunity to improve future standards of practice in the unit concerned, rather than a collective "guilt-trip" or, still worse, a search for a scapegoat.

Some suicides, for example those resulting from an acute severe depressive illness which could almost certainly have been cured, are major tragedies. In other cases, for example those associated with chronic intractable mental or physical illness, the argument for prevention is not so strong. Recent proposals for legalising "medically assisted" suicide have aroused much professional and public controversy.

NON-FATAL DELIBERATE SELF-HARM (DSH, PARASUICIDE, ATTEMPTED SUICIDE)

Definition

Non-fatal deliberate self-harm is deliberate overdose or self-injury without a fatal outcome.

Frequency

Non-fatal deliberate self-harm is at least 10 times more common than completed suicide, though an exact frequency is impossible to determine because milder cases may not be referred to hospital, or even present to health services at all. A major epidemic occurred during the 1960s and 1970s, when self-poisoning became the commonest reason for a young person to be admitted to a medical ward. Rates have declined since that time.

Methods

About 90% are self-poisonings, often by proprietary analgesics such as aspirin or paracetamol, and/or prescribed psychotropic drugs, and often accompanied by alcohol. Others are by violent methods, such as self-laceration.

Epidemiology

- *Age*: highest in the late teens and early twenties.
- *Sex*: twice as common in women.
- *Social conditions*: highest rates are in social classes IV and V, and in inner city areas with a high incidence of social problems.

Causes

- *Psychiatric disorder*:
    - Depressive symptoms   50–60%
    - Alcoholism   10–20%
    - Personality disorder   15–30%
    - None   10–20%

Depressive symptoms usually resolve within a week or two, and seldom amount to major depressive illness.
- *Life events and social difficulties*: about 70% of acts follow a distressing event, usually involving disharmony with another person.

Motives

About 10% of episodes are serious suicide attempts which failed. In other cases the reported motivation is to escape from an intolerable situation or state of mind, an appeal for help, or an attempt to influence another person. Some patients cannot explain their motivation.

Assessment

Before a valid psychosocial assessment can be carried out, the patient must have had time to recover from the immediate effects of the self-harm, for example drowsiness or confusion after an overdose. Three aspects require attention:

- Whether there was *serious suicidal intent*, as indicated by:
  - the subject claiming to have wanted to die and to regret survival
  - a premeditated act preceded by making arrangements for death, leaving a suicide note, and taking precautions against discovery
  - use of a method which the subject believed would be fatal
  - features associated with completed suicide, such as older age, social isolation.
- Whether *psychiatric illness* requiring treatment is present.
- Whether *social problems* are present.

It is not feasible, or necessary, for all cases to be assessed by a psychiatrist. Junior medical staff, nurses and social workers in the general hospital can be trained to identify those patients needing psychiatric referral. Standardised rating scales are available to aid the interview assessment.

Management

From 10 to 20% of cases are judged to need psychiatric hospital admission because of psychiatric illness and/or continuing suicidal intentions. About 60% are judged to need psychiatric and/or social work follow-up as outpatients, but a high proportion fail to keep follow-up appointments.

Acute dilemmas may arise in the general hospital when self-harm patients are brought in but refuse medical treatments such as stomach washout, or suture of lacerations. The Mental Health Act 1983 does not cover administration of medical treatment (as opposed to psychiatric treatment) against the patient's will, however in a life-threatening emergency it is permitted to give this under common law. The chosen course of action should be justified in the case-notes, and full explanations to patients and/or relatives given.

Prognosis

About 20% repeat deliberate self-harm in the subsequent year, 1% die by suicide in the subsequent year (nearly a 100-fold increase over the general population suicide rate), and about 10% die by suicide eventually.

Prevention

Primary preventive strategies are similar to those described above for completed suicide.

Psychiatric treatment, social work and counselling have been evaluated for secondary prevention in people who have already carried out an attempt. Although these interventions do help to reduce psychosocial problems, they have not been shown to reduce the repetition rate for deliberate self-harm.

FURTHER READING

Books

Hawton K, Catalan J (1987) *Attempted Suicide: a Practical Guide to its Nature and Management* (2nd edn). Oxford University Press: Oxford

Review Articles

Appleby L (1992) Suicide in psychiatric patients: risk and prevention. *British Journal of Psychiatry* **161**: 746–758

Hawton K (1987) Assessment of suicide risk. *British Journal of Psychiatry* **150**: 145–153

Murphy BM, Puffet A (1995) Pathways to suicide prevention. *British Journal of Hospital Medicine* **54**: 11–14

Owens D, House A (1995) Assessment of deliberate self-harm. *Advances in Psychiatric Treatment* **1**: 124–130

15
Eating Disorders: Anorexia Nervosa and Bulimia Nervosa

ANOREXIA NERVOSA

Definition

Anorexia nervosa, named by Gull in 1874, is characterised by:

- *Extreme weight loss* (at least 15%) deliberately achieved by dieting and/or other means such as exercise or purgation.
- *Amenorrhoea* in females, *impotence* in males.
- *Abnormal attitudes* to food.
- *Distorted body image*, with a morbid fear of fatness.

Prevalence

About 1% of adolescent girls in the UK have the full syndrome, but milder partial versions are common, and prevalence has increased in recent years.

Epidemiology

- *Age*: most cases start in adolescence, but sometimes onset is before puberty or in adult life.

- *Sex*: 95% are female.
- *Social class*: patients tend to come from families in social classes 1 and 2.
- *Occupation*: occupations which demand a slim figure, for example modelling, beauty therapy and ballet dancing, are over-represented.
- *Nationality*: the condition mostly affects white subjects living in Western countries.

Causes

- *Psychodynamic theories* view anorexia nervosa as a means of avoiding maturation, especially in sexual terms; or as a means of acquiring independence, and/or a sense of achievement, through strict control of diet and weight. These attitudes may stem from disturbed family relationships, which are always evident in the established case, although they could then be the result of the condition rather than its cause.
- *Cultural theories* implicate the social and media pressures urging Western teenage girls to be slim and diet-conscious. For example, published fashion photographs are often stretched lengthwise to make the models look even thinner than they really are.

Common to both these approaches is the idea that the anorexia develops, in response to family or peer influences, in a young person who lacks a secure sense of self.

- *Hormonal imbalance*: hypothalamic dysfunction is always present and is probably secondary to the weight loss, but could be a primary abnormality, as suggested by the occurrence of amenorrhoea as an early symptom.

Clinical Features

A decision by a mildly overweight teenager to go on a slimming diet is a common starting-point for this disorder.

- *Physical*: the patient loses weight by dietary restriction, especially of carbohydrate foods, and sometimes also by self-induced vomiting, taking laxatives or diuretics, and excessive exercising. Amenorrhoea may occur before there has been much loss of weight. Male patients show loss of sexual interest and impotence.

Other common physical features are hypotension, bradycardia, constipation, mild hypothermia, and a growth of downy (lanugo) hair. Vomiting or purging may result in disturbance of fluid and electrolyte balance. Bone fractures secondary to osteoporosis may occur in chronic cases.

- *Mental*: the patient is preoccupied with food and weight, takes pride in dieting, and feels guilty about eating more than small amounts. Most patients do not see themselves as unwell or underweight, but feel active, healthy and fashionably slim. In chronic cases greater insight may develop, often resulting in depression.

Differential Diagnosis

- *Chronic debilitating physical disease* such as cancer, pituitary failure, Addison's disease, TB or AIDS.
- *Psychiatric illness*: depression, schizophrenia, obsessive-compulsive disorder.
- *Hypothalamic* lesions.

Physical Complications

- *Hormonal and biochemical changes*:
  - reduction of sex and thyroid hormone secretion, secondary to hypothalamic and pituitary dysfunction
  - increase of growth hormone and cortisol secretion
  - increased insulin response to glucose loading
  - low basal temperature and impaired temperature regulation
  - low basal metabolic rate
  - high serum cholesterol
  - abnormal liver function tests
  - low serum zinc.
- *CT scan of the brain* may show ventricular and sulcal enlargement. These changes are not immediately reversible with weight gain.
- *Osteoporotic bones* in chronic cases.

Treatment

This is often a chronic relapsing and remitting condition and repeated courses of treatment, including hospital admissions, may be necessary.

- *Physical*: first priorities are restoration of weight and correction of physical complications. Severe cases require inpatient care, and compulsory treatment under the Mental Health Act 1983 is occasionally indicated. Weight gain is best achieved by winning the patient's agreement to eat more, and skilled nurses can usually manage this, though many patients will be uncooperative at first, secretly disposing of food or vomiting. Some units use a behavioural approach in which privileges like watching TV or having visitors are conditional on regular weight gain, but many patients find this coercive and unhelpful.

Drug treatment may include the use of major tranquillisers for agitation, and appropriate specific medication for co-existing psychiatric syndromes such as depression or obsessive-compulsive disorder. If antidepressants are indicated, tricyclics with their appetite-stimulating properties are more appropriate than the SSRIs which can cause weight loss.

- *Psychological treatment* includes cognitive or supportive therapy individually or in groups, and efforts to correct abnormal body image, perhaps with the aid of measurements or photographs. Psychodynamic approaches are usually unhelpful. Family factors must also be addressed, as in the case of a girl aged 16 who developed anorexia after her achievement of 8 out of 9 "A" grades at GCSE was perceived by her family as a failure because of the single "B". She felt that the only thing she could succeed at was the control of her weight.

Prognosis

Recovery is judged by return to normal weight, return of menstruation, and improved psychological and psychosexual adjustment. After five years, about half these patients have recovered fully, and a quarter have improved to some degree. Up to 20% die from suicide, malnutrition or physical complications. Poor prognostic features are a long history, older age of onset, abnormal premorbid personality, poor family relationships and extreme weight loss.

Case Example

A 16-year-old schoolgirl, intelligent but lacking in self-confidence, started to diet after a young man said that her tummy was too fat. The girl was working hard for exams at the time, and her parents were having some marital problems. While eating less and less, she became more and more interested in food and spent much time reading recipe books, and baking cakes for the rest of the family. She slept very little, and would get up early to run for an hour before school. Her weight dropped from 8 to 5 stone within about three months, and eventually her mother insisted on taking her to the doctor because her periods had stopped. The girl refused to talk about her condition or accept any medical treatment; however she agreed to eat a little more within strictly controlled limits, for example taking an extra half-pint of milk and two slices of bread each day.

Her weight gradually increased again over the next few months but it was six years before menstruation resumed. She achieved a professional qualification, and held a responsible job throughout her 20s despite drinking half a bottle of vodka in private every night. The drinking decreased in her early 30s after she married an older man; they had no children. Now aged 50, she has continued to maintain her weight at 47 kg precisely and becomes very anxious if prevented, by circumstances such as going on holiday, from weighing herself twice a day.

BULIMIA NERVOSA

Bulimia nervosa, described by Russell in 1979, is characterised by:

- Powerful and intractable *urges to overeat.*
- Efforts to *avoid the fattening effects of food* by inducing vomiting or abusing purgatives.
- Morbid *fear of fatness.*

Bulimia and anorexia are closely related. Many anorexic patients exhibit bulimic symptoms, and 25–50% of bulimic patients have a past history of anorexia.

Prevalence

Depending on diagnostic criteria, about 1–2% of young women in the UK may be diagnosed as bulimic. Many cases can be successfully concealed because, unlike those with anorexia nervosa, bulimia sufferers look outwardly healthy.

Epidemiology

- *Sex*: most cases are female.
- *Age*: late teens or early 20s.
- *Marital status*: about 25% are married.

Patients tend to be older, more sexually experienced, and more confident and outgoing than those with anorexia nervosa.

Clinical Features

- *Physical*: bouts of eating vast quantities of food (bingeing) occur in response to an uncontrollable psychological urge. Self-induced vomiting often follows such episodes.

  In between binges, most patients follow strict diets and may also abuse purgatives or take excessive exercise, so managing to keep their weight within the normal range.
- *Mental*: preoccupation with food and weight dominates patients' lives, but unlike many with anorexia nervosa, bulimic patients show good insight into their abnormal attitudes and behaviour. Depressive symptoms are common. Some patients abuse alcohol and a subgroup shows impulsive behaviour affecting many aspects of life.

Physical Complications

Vomiting and laxative abuse may result in hypokalaemic hypochloraemic alkalosis; this dangerous complication may lead to cardiac arrhythmias (sometimes fatal), fits and renal damage. Another serious but rare complication is acute dilatation of the stomach. Swollen parotid glands, and dental damage due to frequent vomiting, may develop. Menstrual irregularity, or amenorrhoea, is usual for patients who are not on the contraceptive pill.

Treatment

- *Cognitive-behavioural psychotherapy*, individual or group.
- *Antidepressants*, especially the SSRIs in high dose.

Both these approaches are of proven effectiveness.

Prognosis

Few long-term studies are yet available, but the symptoms often persist for years and mortality from suicide or physical complications may be up to 20%.

OBESITY

Obesity is not classed as a psychiatric disorder, but psychologically driven overeating may contribute to its development, and psychological problems may result from it.

FURTHER READING

Fairburn CG (1990) Bulimia nervosa. *British Medical Journal* **300**: 485–487

Hsu LKG (1988) The outcome of anorexia nervosa: a reappraisal. *Psychological Medicine* **18**: 807–812

Mynors-Wallis LM (1989) Psychological treatment of eating disorders. *British Journal of Hospital Medicine* **41**: 470–475

Patton G (1989) The course of anorexia nervosa. *British Medical Journal* **299**: 139–140

Sharp CW, Freeman CPL (1993) The medical complications of anorexia nervosa. *British Journal of Psychiatry* **162**: 452–462

16

Disorders of Female Reproductive Life

This chapter covers psychiatric disorder in relation to pregnancy, childbirth and motherhood, and the menstrual cycle.

PREGNANCY

Pregnancy appears, broadly speaking, to protect against psychiatric disorder; an effect having probable survival value in evolutionary terms. First onset of psychiatric disorder during pregnancy is rare, existing disorders tend to become less severe, and suicide rates during pregnancy and the puerperium are low.

However, women with a history of chronic or recurrent psychiatric disorder require continuing assessment and care during pregnancy, and monitoring to detect and treat any worsening after childbirth, with the health and safety of both mother and baby in mind.

Psychotropic drug treatment during pregnancy, though best avoided for the baby's sake, is sometimes essential for the mother's mental health. There is no evidence that antipsychotics, tricyclic antidepressants or benzodiazepines cause serious harm to the foetus though, for example, a newborn whose mother had been taking a benzodiazepine might exhibit a transient withdrawal syndrome. Lithium should however be avoided, because it may cause foetal thyroid enlargement and, if taken in the first trimester, foetal cardiac malformation. It is important that the mother receives full information about proposed drug therapy, and gives informed consent (see *British National Formulary* guidelines on prescribing in pregnancy).

ECT can safely be given in pregnancy.

Unplanned pregnancies sometimes occur in women whose judgement is affected by psychiatric illness or learning disability, and may remain undiagnosed until a late stage.

PUERPERAL PSYCHOSIS

Definition

Psychosis beginning within 12 weeks of delivery.

Frequency

After 1 in 500 births.

Predisposing Factors

- Past history of psychosis.
- Family history of psychosis.
- Primiparity.

Causes

- *Medical disorders*: pelvic infections, thromboembolism and other physical complications of childbirth, though not common nowadays, need to be excluded in every case. The classical psychiatric picture is one of delirium but, in early cases, confusion may only be apparent on detailed cognitive testing.
- *Hormone changes*: the abrupt fall in oestrogen and progesterone concentrations which occurs following delivery could precipitate psychosis in predisposed women.
- *Psychosocial stress*: childbirth as a major "life event" could precipitate psychosis in predisposed women.

Clinical Features

Premonitory symptoms may occur in late pregnancy, but onset of frank psychosis is usually sudden, 2–14 days after delivery. Even in the majority of cases which do not have an identified physical cause, symptoms such as confusion, emotional lability and perplexity are often prominent. Depressive and manic syndromes are commoner than schizophrenic ones, though mixed pictures often occur. The thought content, and any delusions or hallucinations present (for example "I am too wicked to be a mother"; "this baby's body is rotting inside") occasionally lead the patient to harm or even kill herself and/or her child.

Treatment

These illnesses can be severe and unpredictable. The safety of the mother and particularly of the baby must always be paramount. Hospital admission is usually necessary, preferably to one of the specialised mother and baby units which exist in some health districts.

Treatment is in principle the same as would be used for the equivalent psychosis occurring apart from the puerperium. However, ECT should more readily be considered, for manic and schizophrenic syndromes as well as depressive ones. ECT often relieves symptoms more quickly than drugs, and most psychotropic drugs enter breast milk which is a potential (though sometimes overemphasised) concern if the mother is breast-feeding. High-dose progesterone is reported to be helpful but has not been tested in a clinical trial. The issue of contraception may need addressing if the illness is at all prolonged.

Prognosis

Short-term prognosis is good, but there is a 20% chance of recurrence after any subsequent pregnancy, and a 50% chance of later recurrence not related to pregnancy.

POSTNATAL NEUROSES

Any neurotic disorder can occur in the postnatal period. In addition to postnatal depression and "maternity blues", the two syndromes most frequently described (see below), anxiety disorders and obsessive-compulsive disorders sometimes occur. Symptomatology usually centres on the baby. Affected mothers often try to hide their symptoms because they know they are expected to be happy at this time, feel ashamed of their negative attitudes towards their babies, or are afraid the babies will be taken into care.

Maternity Blues

About 50% of mothers experience irritability, lability of mood and tearfulness following delivery, maximal at about four days, tending gradually to resolve by about day 10. Such symptoms may be considered normal in the sense of being extremely common; however they can cause considerable distress to the patient and family, and there is evidence of a weak linkage with psychiatric disorder. This is an appropriate subject for prenatal education, and supportive care from family, midwife and GP. If the syndrome fails to resolve, further care may be required.

Postnatal Depression

Depression which is more persistent than "maternity blues" occurs after 10–20% of births. Many cases represent continuation, exacerbation or recurrence of depression which was present before the birth or even before the pregnancy. A subgroup of women suffer depressive illness specifically related to childbirth, and their rates of depression at other times are not raised. Psychological difficulties in adjusting to motherhood, coping with the added responsibilities and changed social role, especially when there are social problems such as lack of support from the child's father or poor housing, may contribute to these depressive states. Minor hormone imbalance might also be involved.

Clinical features are not distinct from other depressive illnesses, and may include depression of mood, anxiety, panic attacks, fatigue, loss of libido, anorexia and insomnia. Some of these symptoms are difficult to distinguish from the inevitable changes in sleep, eating pattern and sexual function brought about by giving birth and caring for a child. Thoughts of hating or wishing to harm the baby are common, and should always sensitively be asked about; the mother will feel very guilty about any thoughts of this kind, and may be much helped by talking about them, and understanding that she is not alone in experiencing them. Actual harming of the baby is rare

---

Case Example

A 29-year-old professional woman lived comfortably with her husband and two small children. Her third pregnancy was unplanned but the couple seemed to accept it well. Mid-way through the pregnancy the husband was made redundant, and they began to experience some marital difficulties. During the third trimester, the patient became increasingly tearful and tired. She had a prolonged and painful labour, but the baby was well and breast-feeding was established satisfactorily.

At home over the next two weeks, the health visitor noticed the patient became very distressed when her baby cried and seemed not to know what to do. She appeared mildly perplexed and was not taking much care of herself or her surroundings. On questioning, she confirmed that she could hardly sleep, had little appetite, her weight was dropping fast and she could not enjoy her baby as she had enjoyed the other two. She admitted feeling "ugly" and "dirty" (because of dribbling milk) and had considered leaving home because she was such a bad mother and wife. She scored 18 (high) on the Edinburgh Postnatal Depression Scale.

The health visitor called the GP, who visited the family and confirmed the diagnosis of depression, prescribed a tricyclic anti-depressant (compatible with breast-feeding), and encouraged the health visitor to offer ongoing supportive counselling in addition to monitoring the baby's well-being.

Within six weeks the patient's mood had lifted and she was restored to her former competent self, returning to work part-time while her husband stayed at home to look after the children. She continued on medication for another six months, during which time the couple came to accept their new circumstances and re-established a good emotional and sexual relationship.

unless the mother is psychotic. The illness may last for months or years especially if, as is often the case, it goes undetected and untreated. This chronic ill-health in the mother is believed to hinder cognitive and emotional development in the child.

Treatment includes a combination of the following:

- *Social support*: training in child care, ongoing contact with named midwives and health visitors, introduction to other mothers of young children. Such measures in pregnancy have been shown to have preventive value, and health visitors given special training can provide valuable supportive counselling after the birth.
- *Antidepressant drugs*.
- *Psychotherapy*: individual, marital, family or group.

ABORTION

The Abortion Act 1967, with its subsequent amendments, permits abortion before 24 weeks' gestation in the case of risk to the mother's life, the mother's physical health or mental health, or the health of her existing children; later abortion is permitted in the case of foetal abnormality. Most abortions are carried out on the grounds of risk to the mother's mental health, but usually without a psychiatric opinion.

Postpartum psychosis after a previous delivery is usually regarded as a justification for abortion if the woman wants one, but since the risk of recurrence of postpartum psychosis after a single previous episode is only 20%, abortion should not necessarily be advised in such cases.

Abortion seldom has serious psychiatric sequelae, but about 25% of women experience significant guilt or depression afterwards, especially if they were ambivalent about the abortion or pressurised to accept it.

STILLBIRTH AND PERINATAL DEATH

Mothers of babies who were stillborn, or died soon after birth, almost always develop grief reactions as found after other forms of bereavement (Ch 5), are at high risk of prolonged depression and have an increased suicide rate. Fathers are also affected but have not been so thoroughly studied. Management after neonatal bereavement should include opportunities for the parents to see and touch the dead child, encouragement to give the baby a name, take a photograph, hold a funeral, receive an explanation for the death and obstetric/genetic advice about future pregnancies, and bereavement counselling from an experienced professional. Such measures have been shown to reduce the duration of psychiatric morbidity.

PREMENSTRUAL SYNDROME

Many women report depressed mood, irritability or anxiety, often combined with physical symptoms such as breast tenderness, headaches, bloated feelings and weight gain, for up to two weeks before the onset of menstruation. Oestrogens by transdermal patches are an effective treatment, so is the SSRI fluoxetine. Many other drug treatments including progesterone, oral contraceptives, diuretics, pyridoxine (B6), bromocriptine and evening primrose oil sometimes seem helpful in individual cases. Premenstrual tension has been used successfully as a defence in criminal trials.

THE MENOPAUSE

Epidemiological studies do not demonstrate any increase in major psychiatric morbidity in women of menopausal age. However, mild to moderate depression or anxiety may develop at this time of life; perhaps secondary to hormone changes, perhaps reactive to physical symptoms, or perhaps reflecting life changes such as children leaving home, death of parents and awareness of ageing. The value of hormone replacement therapy in treating mood disturbance in menopausal women is debated.

HYSTERECTOMY

Depressive reactions may occur following hysterectomy; some women having this operation are distressed by the loss of their childbearing capacity and/or their sense of femininity. However, follow-up of women having hysterectomies for menorrhagia of benign origin shows the majority to be pleased with the results, and overall psychiatric morbidity significantly lower after the operation than before, though still higher than in the general population.

FURTHER READING

Kendell RE (1985) Invited review: emotional and physical factors in the genesis of puerperal mental disorders. *Journal of Psychosomatic Research* **29**: 3–11

Harris B (1994) Biological and hormonal aspects of postpartum depressed mood. *British Journal of Psychiatry* **164**: 288–292

O'Brien PMS (1993) Helping women with premenstrual syndrome. *British Medical Journal* **307**: 1471–1475

Oates M (1995) Risk and childbirth in psychiatry. *Advances in Psychiatric Treatment* **1**: 146–152

Pearce J, Hawton K, Blake F (1995) Psychological and sexual symptoms associated with the menopause and the effects of hormone replacement therapy. *British Journal of Psychiatry* **167**: 163–173

Snaith RP (1983) Pregnancy-related psychiatric disorder. *British Journal of Hospital Medicine* **29**: 450–456

Zolese G, Blacker CVR (1992) The psychological consequences of therapeutic abortion. *British Journal of Psychiatry* **160**: 742–749

17

Sexual Problems

Sexual problems may present in various medical settings: primary care, general or specialist psychiatric practice, gynaecology, urology and genito-urinary medicine (GUM) clinics, also in non-health settings such as Relate (formerly the Marriage Guidance Council). Whether or not certain variants of sexual behaviour or function are perceived as "problems" will depend on the expectations, and moral values, of the individual and of his or her social group. Topics in this chapter are arranged as follows:

- *Sexual dysfunctions*: sexual performance fails to satisfy the subject or partner.
- *Sexual deviations*: sexual practice departs from convention in a way which distresses the subject or offends others.
- *Gender identity disorders*.
- *Homosexuality*, which is not a disorder, but is conveniently considered here.

SEXUAL DYSFUNCTIONS

These conditions, in which some aspect of sexual performance fails to satisfy the subject or partner, may be categorised in several ways but perhaps most clearly by relating them to the five stages in the model of normal sexual response described by Masters and Johnson.

	Male	*Female*
Desire	reduced libido	reduced libido
Excitement	erectile dysfunction	unresponsiveness
Intercourse	loss of erection	vaginismus
Orgasm	premature/delayed ejaculation	anorgasmia
Resolution	priapism	
All stages	dyspareunia	dyspareunia

Reduced libido in women, and erectile and ejaculatory problems in men, are among the most common reasons that couples present for advice. The terms "frigidity" and "impotence" are imprecise and judgemental, and should be avoided.

Causes

- *Background factors*: anxiety or ignorance about sex, past experience of sexual abuse, general disharmony between the couple concerned, a constitutional discrepancy in sex drive between the two partners or a lack of physical attraction between them.
- *Ageing*: sexual drive and performance in both sexes decrease with age, though the decline is more marked in males. For example, the prevalence of erectile dysfunction in men is about 2% at age 40, and 25–30% at age 65.
- *Psychiatric illness*: most psychiatric illnesses, especially depressive illness and anxiety states, reduce sexual drive, performance and pleasure. The exception is mania, in which sexual interest and activity increase.
- *Organic brain disease*: the dementias, and lesions of the frontal lobe, may produce sexual disinhibition.
- *Genital and pelvic pathology*: for example congenital abnormality, infection, injury to the genitalia or spinal cord.
- *Endocrine and metabolic disorders*: for example diabetes, sex hormone deficiency, hyperprolactinaemia, hypertension, arteriosclerosis, renal failure.
- *Drugs*: psychotropic drugs, especially antidepressants and neuroleptics, may affect sexual function and so may many of the drugs used in general medicine, for example antihypertensives and diuretics.
- *Alcohol*: impaired sexual function in male alcoholics may result from intoxication, peripheral neuropathy, disturbed sex hormone

metabolism due to cirrhosis of the liver, marital conflict, or treatment with disulfiram.

Assessment

If both partners attend they should, if they agree, be interviewed separately and then together. The two parties frequently differ in their view of what the problem is, and in their desire for treatment, and it is important to be clear about such differences. The duration of the problem, and whether it is present with other partners and on masturbation, should be established. A medical history, psychiatric history and physical examination should always be obtained, followed by laboratory investigations if indicated. It is especially important to use a sensitive, non-judgemental style when interviewing people with sexual problems.

Treatment

● *Underlying causes* such as psychiatric or medical illness should be managed appropriately.

● *Psychological approaches*: simple explanation and counselling may be all that is required, and sometimes can be best provided from the many useful books and videos available to the public. More complex cases may need formal psychotherapy, individually or as a couple.

● *Sex therapy*: this derives from the methods of Masters and Johnson. The couple are usually treated together. Treatment begins with a "sensate focus" phase during which intercourse is not attempted, so that the couple stop repeating an experience of failure, but spend a set time alone together each day to concentrate on talking about relationship issues and exchanging non-genital physical affection. In stages, the couple then work towards genital stimulation, followed by intercourse. They may be taught specific techniques according to the type of dysfunction present, for example the "squeeze technique" for premature ejaculation, or extended foreplay in orgasmic delay.

Case Example

A man aged 52, happily married for 23 years, was referred to psychiatric outpatients by his GP who said his patient was distressed by "progressive impotence", and had recently watched a television programme about "penile injection treatment" which he was keen to try. The man himself seemed rather embarrassed by the referral. He attended without his wife, and had not told her about it; she had "not seemed especially keen on sex" after the menopause, and they had been having intercourse about every two weeks in recent years, largely at his request. He had recently taken an antihypertensive drug, and had been finding it more difficult to sustain an erection; although his blood pressure had since settled and he was able to stop this medication, his erectile difficulty had not entirely resolved. Direct inquiry established that there was less of a problem during masturbation.

The psychiatrist could detect no physical or mental disorder, and blood tests including prolactin were normal. He advised that the problem would probably continue to resolve, and that specific treatment was not required at present, though a course of tablets (yohimbine) was available if necessary in the future.

At follow-up, the patient was invited to ask his wife to attend. There had been some further improvement in his erections, but it emerged that his underlying fear was that he was "failing in his marital duties". The psychiatrist advised that their sexual relationship, in particular their frequency of intercourse, was entirely normal for their age. Although it was possible that the wife was suffering from some oestrogen deficiency symptoms including vaginal dryness, which might well have responded to hormone replacement therapy, the couple declined further appointments, saying they were "reasonably happy with things as they are".

- *Systemic drugs*: these are appropriate when a specific medical indication is present. Examples include:
  - oestrogen/progesterone hormone replacement therapy in postmenopausal women
  - yohimbine tablets (available on a named-patient basis) in erectile dysfunction

- androgen treatment for reduced sexual drive in men who have low testosterone levels
- certain antidepressants (trazodone, SSRIs) for erectile failure
- bromocriptine for male sexual dysfunction secondary to hyperprolactinaemia.

- *Local treatments for female partner*:
  - topical lubricants/oestrogens for vaginal dryness
  - vaginal dilators, of progressively larger size, for vaginismus.
- *Local treatments for males with erectile failure*:
  - intracavernosal injection of vasoactive drugs such as papaverine, prostaglandin E1 (aprostadil)
  - topical vasodilators such as nitrates
  - vacuum devices, using suction to establish erection which is then maintained by a ring
  - surgical implants.

Prognosis

About 30% of clients treated at sex therapy clinics improve a great deal and a further 30% show some improvement.

SEXUAL DEVIATIONS

Most variants of sexual orientation and behaviour, sometimes called "paraphilias" or "alternative sexual practices", are no longer classed as psychiatric disorders, and more liberal attitudes in society during recent years have reduced the frequency of psychiatric involvement with them. However, sometimes these variants are associated with psychiatric disorder, social maladjustment, or transgressions of the law. Psychiatric treatment is only indicated when a sexual deviation leads to suffering for the subject or for other people, and only with the subject's willing consent.

Causes

The cause of sexual deviations is generally unknown. These conditions, which are much commoner in males than females, usually present by early adulthood or before. They may therefore be regarded as a permanent feature of the personality which may become more marked with the passage of years or at times of stress. Some of these behaviours are associated with difficulty in forming normal relationships, for example indecent exposure may occur in men with poor social skills and/or learning disability. Availability is also a factor, for example bestiality among men with ready access to animals. There may be a genetic component. In rare cases, first onset in later life appears due to functional psychiatric illness or organic brain disease.

Psychodynamic theorists have suggested these behaviours are due to abnormal parental attitudes, for example excessive dominance of one parent, or parental desire for a child of the opposite sex. In the behavioural model, deviant sexual behaviour is conceived as being learned by conditioning or modelling, and maintained by reward in the form of orgasm and anxiety reduction.

Individual deviations will now be described.

Sadism and Masochism

Sadism is sexual gratification from inflicting cruelty on the partner. Masochism, which often co-exists in the same individual, is sexual gratification from being subjected to cruelty. Minor forms of both conditions are common. Extreme forms of sadism can lead to sexual crimes.

Fetishism

A group of conditions in which sexual desire is focused on a body part other than the genitals (for example the feet) or an inanimate object (for example a particular type of garment). If treatment is indicated at all, behaviour therapy is the treatment of choice.

Bestiality

Bestiality is intercourse with animals, most common among male farm workers. It is illegal.

Indecent Exposure

Indecent exposure (exhibitionism) is illegal exposure of the genitals to another person, usually carried out by a man in the presence of a girl or woman who is unknown to him. Most exhibitionists are young men who expose a flaccid penis; these are anxious, inhibited personalities whose sexual adjustment is poor, and feel guilty about exposing. They often cease the behaviour after detection. A minority are sociopathic men who expose an erect penis whilst masturbating, and derive pleasure and excitement from the act. This group is more likely to repeat the behaviour, and to progress to more serious offences.

Paedophilia

Paedophilia is a sexual preference for children. Sexual contact with a child under 16 is an imprisonable offence. Most cases involve men, and less often women, who have difficulty forming sexual relationships with adults. Many have themselves been abused as children. Homosexual and heterosexual types exist. Behaviour ranges from an affectionate relationship with a known child to the homicidal rape of a strange one. Dangerous paedophiliacs require secure care and antilibidinal drugs. See also Child Sexual Abuse (Ch 18).

Incest

Incest is sexual intercourse with a parent, sibling, child or grandchild, and is an imprisonable offence. The most common forms are between father and daughter, and between brother and sister. It is often associated with social deprivation and overcrowding, and/or a poor sexual relationship between the parents in the family. Some girls involved in incestuous relationships have sexual difficulties in later life, but the frequency of long-term ill-effects is unknown. There is a greatly increased risk of genetic defects in children conceived through incest. See also Child Sexual Abuse (Ch 18).

Rape is considered in Ch 21.

Treatment

● *Behavioural and cognitive therapy*: older techniques such as aversion therapy were designed to discourage unwanted desires and behaviours, but are now little used because of ethical objections. Modern approaches place greater emphasis on positive conditioning by encouraging preferable alternatives. For example, paedophilia may be treated with "orgasmic reconditioning" in which, during masturbation, the subject is encouraged to concentrate on acceptable fantasies. For deviations which appear to be a substitute for adult heterosexual relationships, in men who lack confidence about approaching women, assertiveness or social skills training may help.
● *Group therapy* is often used for offenders, who are thereby encouraged to confront the effects of their behaviour on victims.
● *Drugs*: antilibidinal drugs for male sexual offenders include the anti-androgen *cyproterone acetate*, the major tranquilliser *benperidol*, *oestrogens*, and the gonadorelin analogue *goserilin*. These drugs may cause impotence, infertility and breast enlargement, so they should only be used for dangerous sex offenders and (as laid down in the Mental Health Act 1983) only with the support of two approved consultant psychiatrists' opinions plus the subject's own informed consent.
● *Psychodynamic psychotherapy* to explore possible origins of the sexual deviation in disturbed relationships or repressed events in childhood.

Few of the above treatments have been rigorously demonstrated to be effective, and it is particularly important to remember this in forensic cases. Therapeutic optimism has led to some recidivist sexual offenders being removed from the criminal justice system into the healthcare system, and subsequent re-offending wrongly attributed by the media to failures of psychiatric care rather than the elective behaviour of the offender. Some sex offenders feign a wish for psychiatric help because they hope to avoid a prison sentence.

Castration for sex offenders is not allowed in the UK even if the subject requests it.

GENDER IDENTITY DISORDERS

Transvestism

Transvestism is a wish or compulsion to wear clothing of the opposite sex. Most transvestites are male, and most are heterosexual, but sometimes the condition is associated with homosexuality, transsexualism or sexual deviations. Transvestism is common and not illegal.

Transsexualism

Transsexualism is a rare disorder of sexual identity in which there is a strong wish to change to the opposite sex, with a belief of having been born into the wrong sex, present since early childhood. Most subjects are biologically male. Many are married men with children, but a few are homosexual.

Transsexuals usually present for treatment because they want surgical sex reassignment. Most reputable practitioners will only carry out such operations if the subject has received thorough information and counselling, successfully lived in the role of the opposite sex for two years with the aid of hormone therapy, is currently unmarried, and free of psychiatric disorder. Most subjects who fulfil these criteria are pleased with the results of surgery. The male-to-female operation, involving removal of the penis and scrotum and creation of an artificial vagina, is more satisfactory than the female-to-male version and should enable the subject to experience sexual intercourse as a woman (but not, of course, to bear children as a few naïve subjects expect). The operation is combined with breast surgery, ongoing hormone treatment to change the secondary sex characteristics, and tuition in behaviour appropriate to the new sex. In law, the sex remains the original one as stated on the birth certificate and therefore subjects cannot legally marry in their new role.

HOMOSEXUALITY

Homosexuality, an exclusive or predominant sexual preference for the same sex, is no longer classed as a psychiatric disorder. It is mentioned here because it may be associated with increased rates of depression, alcoholism and neurosis, probably because of the associated social stigma. Social attitudes towards male homosexuality have become well publicised since the advent of HIV and AIDS.

Male homosexual acts are not illegal provided they are carried out in private between consenting males both over the age of 21.

Homosexual interests or experiences are common in adolescence. According to community surveys, up to 4% of adult males are exclusively homosexual (gay) and an additional minority of men are bisexual to some degree. The percentages for females are similar.

Some homosexuals resemble the opposite sex in their physical habits, mannerisms or dress.

Causation of homosexuality, like heterosexuality, remains unclear. Reported biological factors include a genetic component as demonstrated by twin studies, and an X-linked gene in some male homosexuals has recently been reported. No consistent abnormalities of sex hormone secretion have been found, although hormone imbalance in the prenatal period has been suggested. Psychodynamic factors, for example the combination of a doting mother and weak or absent father, have also been implicated. Bancroft's 1994 review concluded that "it remains difficult, on scientific grounds, to avoid the conclusion that the uniquely human phenomenon of sexual orientation is a consequence of a multifactorial developmental process in which biological factors play a part, but in which psychosocial factors remain crucially important".

In the past, various interventions including psychotherapy, behaviour therapy and hormone treatments were tried in order to modify homosexual orientation, all to little effect. This is no longer considered appropriate, and modern approaches are designed to aid adaptation to the homosexual state, with any co-existing psychiatric disorder being treated in standard fashion. For homosexuals facing other difficulties, services organised by gays themselves, such as telephone advice and self-help groups, are appropriate sources of support.

FURTHER READING

Books

Bancroft J (1990) *Human Sexuality and its Problems* (2nd edn). Churchill Livingstone (Longman Group): London
Delvin D (1992) *The Book of Love*. Hodder-Headline: London

Review Articles

Bancroft J (1994) Homosexual orientation. *British Journal of Psychiatry* **164**: 437–440

Friedman RC, Downey JI (1994) Homosexuality. *New England Journal of Medicine* **331**: 923–930

Hawton K (1983) Behavioural approaches to the management of sexual deviations. *British Journal of Psychiatry* **143**: 248–255

Hawton K (1995) Treatment of sexual dysfunctions by sex therapy and other approaches. *British Journal of Psychiatry* **167**: 307–314

Kirby RS (1994) Impotence: diagnosis and management of male erectile dysfunction. *British Medical Journal* **308**: 957–961

18
Child and Adolescent Psychiatry

Child and adolescent psychiatrists deal with patients up to school-leaving age.

Most psychiatric disorders of childhood involve a quantitative rather than qualitative abnormality of emotion, conduct or rate of development. Emotions or conduct considered abnormal at one age may be normal at another.

Community surveys have indicated that between 7% and 20% of children can be diagnosed as having psychiatric disorder. Prevalence is higher in inner city areas than rural ones. Only about 10% of affected children receive psychiatric treatment.

Before puberty, boys have more psychiatric disorder than girls, and conduct disorders are more common than emotional disorders. During adolescence the rates increase, with more girls affected and a higher proportion of emotional disorders.

PREDISPOSING FACTORS

Most cases probably have a multifactorial causation, including genetic predisposition to psychiatric disorder; biological factors such as poor nutrition before and/or after birth; and a psychologically stressful and/or deprived environment. Individual factors associated with childhood psychiatric disorder include:

- Organic brain disease.
- Chronic physical disease.
- Low intelligence.
- Child abuse (see below).
- Discord within the family, and undesirable parental attitudes which include overprotection as well as hostility or neglect.
- Physical or mental illness in another family member, especially the mother. In the case of psychiatric disorder, the child's mental health may be at risk because of genetic factors as well as disruption to the home environment.
- Separation from the mother, especially if there is no adequate substitute. Bowlby's work on maternal deprivation formed the basis of "attachment theory", emphasising the importance of a consistent caregiver, who is usually but not necessarily the biological mother, during early life.
- Adoption.
- Single parent family.
- Lower social class.
- Poverty.
- Antisocial behaviour in family.
- Large family.
- Ethnic minority.

CLASSIFICATION

In clinical practice disorders are usually grouped as follows:

- Emotional/neurotic disorders.
- Conduct disorders.
- Psychoses.
- Specific delays in development.
- Symptomatic.

It is useful to consider a *multiaxial* approach, including:

- Clinical psychiatric syndrome.
- Developmental level.
- Intellectual level.
- Medical conditions.
- Psychosocial situation.

HISTORY-TAKING AND EXAMINATION

The child and both parents (or other main carers) need to be interviewed, either together or separately depending on the age of the child and the preferences of those concerned. Most of the history has to be obtained from the parents if the child is young. A separate interview with the parents may reveal problems of their own which are affecting the child, or have arisen through living with a disturbed child.

History

- *Complaint.*
- *History of present difficulties.*
- *Family*: age, occupation, mental and physical health of parents and siblings. A personal history of the parents including their own childhood. Emotional atmosphere of the household.
- *Developmental history*:
  - pregnancy; whether planned, obstetric complications
  - milestones
  - illnesses
  - separations from parents, and reactions to these.
- *School*: academic achievements, relations with other children and with teachers.
- *Life events* and *social difficulties*.

Interview with Child

The older the child, the more he or she will be able to give a direct account of the problems. Although information from younger children may have to be obtained indirectly through play, drawing, asking the child to tell a story or give "three wishes", direct inquiry about the problems as perceived by the child should never be omitted.

Mental State

Observation of mental state is carried out under the same headings used in adult psychiatry. Particular attention should be given to signs suggesting minor neurological impairment: over- or underactivity, poor coordination, short attention span.

Physical Examination

Neurological examination should be included.

Psychological Testing

This may be done by the educational psychology service provided by local authorities to schools, or by the health service, and includes:

- Intelligence.
- Educational achievements.
- Personality assessment.
- Motor and perceptual development.

Independent Informant

- Schoolteacher.
- Social worker.
- General practitioner/health visitor.

A telephone call to a professional with knowledge of the family will frequently clarify a problem impossible to sort out in the consulting room.

TREATMENT

Psychological therapies, whether using a psychodynamic approach or a cognitive-behavioural one, have traditionally predominated over drug treatments in child psychiatry. The whole family should preferably be involved in therapy, since family functioning appears to have a marked influence on most psychiatric disorders of childhood. Sometimes, though the child is presented as the patient, the primary problem turns out to lie with another family member, for example a mother who is suffering from depression. In other cases, parents or siblings are being secondarily affected by the child's emotional disturbance.

Child psychiatry is usually practised in the community, and inpatient admission is rare. In child and family therapy centres, a team of professionals including child psychiatrists, educational psychologists, social workers, child psychotherapists and community nurses carry out multidisciplinary treatment. Child psychiatrists and their colleagues also practise in general hospitals, special schools, social services assessment units and remand homes.

Both assessment and management require collaboration between health, education, social and legal services. Liaison child psychiatry is concerned with physically ill children, both in hospital and community settings.

RELATIONSHIP WITH ADULT DISORDER

Prospective follow-up studies indicate that children with conduct disorders often continue to behave antisocially in adult life. Neurotic disorders have a better prognosis, but are weakly associated with adult neurosis of the same type. Childhood psychosis has a poor long-term outcome.

Retrospective studies of adults with major mental illness, schizophrenia and bipolar affective disorder show an excess of both conduct and neurotic disorders in childhood. However, only a minority of emotionally disturbed children will develop major mental illness when they grow up.

The main clinical syndromes will now be described.

NEUROTIC (EMOTIONAL) DISORDERS

Classical forms of neurotic illness such as anxiety states or obsessive-compulsive disorders sometimes occur in childhood, but mixed syndromes are more usual. Isolated phobias and rituals are common in otherwise well-adjusted children.

School Attendance Problems

School refusal is reluctance to attend school, either due to fear of teachers or other children (school phobia), or fear of leaving the mother (separation anxiety). The mother often covertly encourages it because she herself is depressed or immature, and reluctant to be separated from the child. The child may complain of headache or abdominal pain on school mornings. Treatment includes psychotherapy for the child and mother, dealing with any contributory factors at school, and encouragement to attend.

School refusal should be distinguished from *truanting*, which is staying away from school to do something more enjoyable, and is classed as a conduct disorder.

Affective Disorders

Depression: depressive symptoms, often reactive to a loss or other life stress, are common in young children but the full-blown picture of depressive illness is rare before puberty. Somatic symptoms like anorexia, abdominal pain or headaches are a frequent presentation. Psychotherapy and/or antidepressant drugs are often used, although several clinical trials suggest that antidepressants are no more effective than placebo in this age group.

Bipolar affective disorder occasionally starts in childhood, with either depressive or manic episodes. *Mania* may be misdiagnosed as conduct disorder or hyperkinetic syndrome (see below).

Suicide in early childhood is rare but suicide in adolescents, especially males, is increasing.

CONDUCT DISORDERS

Conduct disorders involve persistent antisocial behaviour: stealing, lying, vandalism, truancy, aggression, sexual disturbances. They are associated with adverse social circumstances, and with brain damage, and are about four times more common in boys than in girls. Treatment involves social casework and/or psychotherapy, family therapy being increasingly used. Behaviour therapy may modify a circumscribed problem.

Delinquency

"Juvenile delinquency" is law-breaking behaviour in children over the age of 10. Delinquency is strongly associated with social factors: disturbed families, large families, criminality in other family members, poverty, residence in certain city neighbourhoods. In some areas, about 20% of boys show delinquent behaviour. Delinquency is also associated with individual factors: low intelligence, brain damage, and minor physical deformities. Management of serious cases may involve supervision by a probation officer, local authority care or a period of community service, but it is uncertain whether such measures influence the outcome. About 40% of persistently delinquent teenagers become criminals in adult life.

ATTENTION DEFICIT DISORDER

Attention deficit disorder (hyperkinetic syndrome) is characterised by restlessness, impulsiveness, inability to concentrate and short attention span. It is more common in boys. There is often a history of birth trauma, or other cerebral insult in early life. Aggressive behaviour, low intelligence, epilepsy, minor motor abnormalities and minor EEG changes are sometimes present. Food additives, as in coloured sweets or drinks, may exacerbate the symptoms.

This is a real syndrome but it has tended to be over-diagnosed, especially in the USA, with the term "minimal brain dysfunction" being applied to cases with no demonstrable abnormalities on examination or investigation.

Differential diagnosis includes mania.

A behavioural modification programme combined with special teaching methods at school is the treatment of choice. Avoiding food additives may be helpful. The most effective drug treatment is, paradoxically, with a cerebral stimulant such as dextroamphetamine, methylphenidate or pemoline. These drugs have many adverse effects, including stunting growth, and they may be addictive, so are best reserved for occasional use. Other drugs including haloperidol, tricyclic antidepressants, caffeine and primidone have also been used.

Spontaneous improvement by adolescence is usual.

PSYCHOSES

Childhood psychosis is rare, affecting 40 per 100 000 children. Types include:

Disintegrative (developmental) psychosis: a child between two and eight years, previously normal, becomes emotionally withdrawn, loses speech, deteriorates intellectually, and shows emotional and behavioural disturbance. *Schilder's disease, lipoidoses,* and *SSPE* (subacute sclerosing panencephalitis, due to the measles virus) are among the causes of this rare condition.

Schizophrenia occasionally starts in childhood.

Autism is believed to be associated with abnormalities of cerebellar and brainstem function. Twin studies suggest a genetic predisposition. Prevalence is 20 per 100 000 children, and it is more common in boys. Learning disability, often due to a specific cause such as rubella, is present in 70% of cases whereas parental intelligence is in the normal range. Neurological impairments are found in 25%, and 30% develop epilepsy during adolescence.

Symptoms start within the first 30 months of life and include abnormal response to sound, failure to understand speech, either mutism or abnormal forms of speech (echolalia, nominal aphasia, pronoun reversal), aloofness from people, and insistence on rituals and routines.

Autism seldom recovers and affected children often need institutional care, though their life expectancy is normal. The lower the IQ the worse the prognosis. Special education, behavioural methods and psychotropic drug treatment may produce some improvement.

Kanner's syndrome is autism with a normal IQ.

Asperger's syndrome, or schizoid personality of childhood, may be a mild form of autism and comprises eccentric isolated behaviour with circumscribed interests and stilted speech: "autistic traits".

DELAYS IN DEVELOPMENT

Educational Underachievement

Causes include:

- *Low IQ.*
- *Specific delays in development. Specific reading retardation* or *dyslexia* is an isolated difficulty in learning to read and write, more common in boys and sometimes associated with clumsiness and conduct disorder. *Specific arithmetical disorder* and *specific motor retardation* are also described as isolated syndromes. These disabilities may be improved by special teaching methods.
- *Physical handicaps*: defective vision or hearing, epilepsy.
- *Poor relationships* with parents or teachers, or low parental expectations.
- *Boredom* in bright children.
- *Drug or solvent use.*

Nocturnal Enuresis (Bedwetting)

Bedwetting is a common problem, present in 15% of 5 year olds and 10% of 10 year olds and a small proportion of teenagers. Causes include:

- *Slow maturation*, which may have a genetic component, and is most common in boys from large and socially disadvantaged families.
- *Emotional disturbance.*
- *Medical disorders* such as urinary infection, diabetes.
- *Physical malformation* of the urinary tract.

Treatment is best directed towards the cause. Symptomatic measures include:

- *Practical: limiting fluids* before bed, *toileting* before bed and *lifting* the child at night.
- *Token economy regimes* such as a "star chart" to reward dry nights.
- *Buzzer and pad* device.
- *Tricyclic antidepressants*, effective because of their anticholinergic properties. Imipramine syrup is often used.
- *Desmopressin* nasal spray.

Encopresis (Faecal incontinence)

Bowel control is normally achieved by the age of four years. Faecal incontinence affects 1% of school age children. Causes include:

- *Constipation with overflow* due to physical disorders such as anal fissure, Hirchsprung's disease.
- *Diarrhoea*, due to infection or other physical causes, or anxiety.
- *Psychological problems* such as neurotic disorders or disturbed family relationships.
- *Learning disability.*

SYMPTOMATIC DISORDERS

Tics, and Gilles de la Tourette Syndrome

A tic is a repetitive, purposeless movement such as blinking or grunting, partly under voluntary control. Tics may develop in normal children, and are exacerbated by emotional disturbance. They are best ignored, and usually disappear spontaneously, but if not then behaviour therapy may help.

Gilles de la Tourette syndrome comprises multiple tics and compulsive utterances. Tics first affect the facial muscles, then spread to other parts of the body. Involuntary utterances then occur, barking noises at first, later obscene words or short phrases (coprolalia). Echolalia and echopraxia may be present. Onset is usually in childhood, and boys are affected three times more often than girls. The syndrome has a genetic component, and may be associated with organic brain disease or the presence of minor neurological signs. Medication with haloperidol, pimozide or clonidine, and/or behaviour therapy, may be effective.

Eating Disorders

Anorexia is usually the result of physical ill-health. Excessive parental concern about food can result in anorexia, or lead the child to use food refusal or vomiting to manipulate the parents. Depression is another cause. *Anorexia nervosa* (Ch 15) occasionally affects prepubertal children but more often starts in adolescence.

Overeating is often a compensation for emotional deprivation. Overeating in adolescence usually causes obesity (and hence further emotional difficulties), but this is not always so in younger children, who may remain undersized: "deprivational dwarfism".

"Pica" is eating the inedible. Exploration of objects with the mouth is normal up to two years of age, but may continue for years in children who are blind, have learning disability or lack environmental stimulation. Sucking lead-painted objects may cause mental and physical damage.

CHILD ABUSE

Abuse of children may be physical, sexual and/or emotional. In recent years there has been increased awareness of child abuse, and its actual frequency may also have increased. Up to 5% of children are reported to professional agencies because of suspected abuse.

Most child abuse is carried out by the parents. Such parents are typically young, immature, poor, and were abused during their own childhood. A small minority are mentally ill. There is a raised incidence of factors likely to impair bonding between parents and child: unwanted pregnancy, complications during pregnancy or birth, separations between parents and child, and ill-health in the child.

Physical Abuse (Non-accidental Injury, Baby Battering)

Fractured bones, periosteal haemorrhage, bruises, retinal haemorrhage and cigarette burns are common manifestations. The child is often retarded in both mental and physical development. The parents themselves may bring the child for treatment, claiming the injury was accidental. Some cases lead to the death of the child.

A variant is the *Munchausen syndrome by proxy* in which a carer, usually the mother, fabricates illness in a child by giving a false medical history and/or inflicting deliberate physical harm.

Sexual Abuse

This is a topical and controversial subject. Sexual abuse of children appears to be a common problem, but poses diagnostic difficulties because it is so often concealed. Both over- and underdiagnosis may have serious consequences for both victim and perpetrator. Possibly about 10% of children undergo sexual abuse, ranging from genital fondling to full sexual intercourse.

Most victims are girls, abused by their fathers, brothers, or other male relatives. Sexual abuse of boys is more often carried out by men outside the family, either an authority figure such as teacher, clergyman or scoutmaster, or a stranger who offers bribes. Occasionally the perpetrator is female.

Some cases come to light because the child, or mother, seeks help directly from a treatment agency. More often the presentation is indirect, for example genital bruising or infection; early teenage pregnancy; a crisis like an overdose or running away from home; vague neurotic symptoms or inhibited development. Many cases remain concealed.

Victims of child sex abuse appear to be at increased risk for certain psychiatric disorders in adult life. These include psychosexual difficulties, neuroses, personality disorders, eating disorders, somatisation and deliberate self-harm. The proportion of victims who suffer serious long-term effects of this kind is not known; however most authorities agree that sexual experience with adults is almost always harmful to the child. Even if it takes place in the context of an affectionate relationship, the surrounding secrecy and coercion are likely to induce fear or guilt in the child.

Emotional Abuse and Neglect

Children whose parents are habitually critical and rejecting, and neglectful of physical and/or emotional care, may present with delays in development, recurrent minor physical ailments, or disordered behaviour.

Management of Abuse

Medical assessment of suspected cases of physical or sexual abuse should only be carried out by a consultant paediatrician or child psychiatrist with relevant experience, because of the sensitive nature of this work, and the diagnostic difficulties which may arise. A suspected case should be referred to social services and/or the police.

Social services departments are responsible for prevention and management, and keep a register of children at risk. A conference about any suspected or confirmed case is held, attended by social workers and other professionals such as police, health visitor, GP, paediatrician, child psychiatrist. Under the Children Act (1989) the child's interests should receive priority over any other considerations.

Close surveillance combined with family and individual psychotherapy may enable the family to remain intact but in some cases it is necessary to remove the perpetrator to prison and/or take the abused child into care.

See also Incest and Paedophilia, Ch 17.

PSYCHIATRY OF ADOLESCENCE

Psychiatric disorder is present in 15–20% of adolescents. "Adolescent turmoil" (identity crisis), when the process of maturation involves extreme mood swings, rebellious behaviour or experimentation with contrasting lifestyles, is a common phenomenon which may be confused with psychiatric illness.

Schizophrenia, affective disorders, neuroses, eating disorders, substance misuse and deliberate self-harm may all begin during adolescence, and personality disorders become clearly evident at this time. Drug misuse and completed suicide in adolescents are becoming increasingly common.

Distinguishing adolescents with formal psychiatric illness from those whose problems stem from disturbance of adjustment and relationships, or substance misuse, can require prolonged observation.

Treatment of seriously disturbed adolescents may be carried out in a residential unit. Length of stay is usually several months and treatment methods are predominantly psychotherapeutic, whether or not involving the patient's family.

FURTHER READING

Books

Barker P (1995) *Basic Child Psychiatry* (6th edn). Blackwell Scientific Publications: Oxford

Black D, Cottrell D (1993) *Seminars in Child and Adolescent Psychiatry.* Gaskell: London

Garralda ME (ed) (1993) *Managing Children with Psychiatric Problems.* BMJ Books: London

Graham PJ (1991) *Child Psychiatry: a developmental approach.* Oxford University Press: Oxford

Meadow R (ed) (1989) *ABC of Child Abuse.* BMJ Books: London

Steinberg D (1988) *Basic Adolescent Psychiatry.* Blackwell Scientific Publications: Oxford

Review Articles

Angold A (1988) Childhood and adolescent depression I: Epidemiological and aetiological aspects. *British Journal of Psychiatry* **152**: 601–617

Angold A (1988) Childhood and adolescent depression II: Research in clinical populations. *British Journal of Psychiatry* **153**: 476–492

Cottrell D, Worrall A (1995) Liaison child and adolescent psychiatry. *Advances in Psychiatric Treatment* **1**: 78–85

Glaser D (1991) Treatment issues in child abuse. *British Journal of Psychiatry* **159**: 769–771

Jones D (1996) Management of the sexually abused child. *Advances in Psychiatric Treatment* **2**: 39–45

Prior MR (1987) Biological and neuropsychological approaches to childhood autism. *British Journal of Psychiatry* **150**: 8–17

Robertson MM (1989) The Gilles de la Tourette syndrome: the current status. *British Journal of Psychiatry* **154**: 147–169

Taylor EA (1986) Childhood hyperactivity. *British Journal of Psychiatry* **149**: 562–573

Thompson AE, Kaplan CA (1996) Childhood emotional abuse. *British Journal of Psychiatry* **168**: 143–148

Werry JS (1992) Child psychiatric disorders: are they classifiable? *British Journal of Psychiatry* **161**: 472–480

19

Learning Disability

The terms *learning disability* or *learning difficulties* are now used in preference to older ones such as *mental handicap, mental retardation* or *mental subnormality*. *Mental impairment* is the term used in the Mental Health Act 1983 (Ch 27) to describe the subgroup of patients in whom learning disability co-exists with "abnormally aggressive or seriously irresponsible conduct".

For practical purposes, learning disability is defined in terms of social incompetence and behavioural problems as well as IQ (intelligence quotient) test results. Corresponding IQ levels are about 50–69 for mild cases, and below 49 for severe ones, but many people with IQs below 70 can lead independent lives and do not need special medical or social care.

FREQUENCY

An IQ below 70 is found in 2.5% of the general population, and 0.4% have an IQ below 50. Severe learning disability is 25% more common in males than females, mostly due to X-linked conditions.

CAUSES

About 70% of mild cases belong to the "non-specific" or "subcultural" group, in which handicap results from a poor genetic intellectual endowment combined with a physically, educationally and/or emotionally deprived upbringing. Mild learning disability is associated with poverty, overcrowding, large family size and family disruption. Child abuse (Ch 18) is an important but often unrecognised factor.

About 30% of mild cases, and nearly all severe cases, result from a specific organic pathology. About 35% of severe cases have a gene or chromosome abnormality, Down's syndrome being most frequent, and about 65% have acquired brain damage.

Specific causes can be classified as follows:

- *Chromosome or gene abnormalities*, for example Down's syndrome, phenylketonuria.
- *Primary maldevelopments of the brain of obscure aetiology*, such as spina bifida with hydrocephalus, microgyria.
- *Prenatal factors affecting the mother*, such as rubella, cytomegalovirus, toxoplasmosis, syphilis, radiation, malnutrition, alcoholism, teratogenic drugs.
- *Perinatal damage*, for example birth trauma, anoxia, rhesus incompatibility, extreme prematurity.
- *Postnatal damage*, for example encephalitis, meningitis, lead poisoning, head injury.

DIAGNOSIS AND ASSESSMENT

Severe cases are usually obvious from infancy, because developmental retardation and physical abnormalities are present.

Mild cases may remain undetected until learning difficulties become apparent at school. Differential diagnosis includes deafness and emotional disturbance.

Investigation should be aimed towards finding the cause and effects of the learning disability, and of any associated psychiatric disorder. It includes a medical history, family history, physical examination, mental state examination, chromosome studies, and testing of blood and urine for abnormal metabolites. Discovery of a specific cause enables genetic counselling for the family, and occasionally permits specific treatment for the child, such as special diets for certain enzyme defects. Even if no specific cause is found, a detailed psychological, medical and social assessment will permit informed decisions on aims and methods of management.

ASSOCIATED PHENOMENA

- *Physical defects*: including motor disorders, malformations, impairments of sight and hearing, are present in about 30% of severe cases.
- *Epilepsy*: in about 25%, being more frequent the lower the IQ.
- *Psychiatric illness*: in about 40%. Patients seldom have the linguistic ability to describe psychiatric symptoms, so they present with behaviour disturbance.
- *Behaviour disturbance.* Causes include:
  - a manifestation of the underlying brain damage
  - a manifestation of the underlying genotype (behavioural phenotype)
  - psychiatric illness
  - physical illness
  - excessive, insufficient or inappropriate medication (psychotropics, anticonvulsants)
  - frustration with a boring or repressive environment
  - communication difficulties
  - adjustment reactions following stressful events, for example change of residence or bereavement. People with learning disability may be just as much affected by such psychological stresses as anyone else, and also may need a longer time to adjust to them.

Behaviour disturbance in the form of aggression, overactivity or self-mutilation is present in about half of severe cases, and is often the reason for families requesting institutional care for a child with learning disability. Behaviour disturbance is also found in adults with milder impairments who are living in the community, and often leads to conflict with the law.

Failure to learn desirable behaviour of which the patient is potentially capable, such as speech and self-care, may also be considered as a type of behaviour disturbance.

MANAGEMENT

A multidisciplinary approach is appropriate, with a view to helping people with learning disabilities to integrate into the general community ("normalisation") and achieve fulfilment of such personal needs as close relationships and appropriate occupation.

Medical management includes diagnosis and treatment of physical and psychiatric problems. Methods of assessment and treatment may need to be modified from those used for people without intellectual impairment, and this requires specialist knowledge. If psychotropic drugs are used, the optimum regime has to be found by titrating the dose against the target behaviour, perhaps over a period of several months.

Psychologists are involved in assessing patients' overall intelligence, and any specific defects or abilities. They help to plan individual behavioural treatments, which can be useful even in severe cases for teaching self-care, practical skills and social behaviour. Desirable behaviour or the acquisition of skills is given positive reinforcement by a tangible reward or approving attention. Undesirable behaviour may be a means of seeking attention, in which case it is best ignored, or it can be managed by occupying the patients with interesting alternative activities.

Social and educational aspects are important. Improving the environment of children from deprived backgrounds has been shown to lead to increases in IQ, though it is uncertain whether this improvement is maintained into adult life. Many parents of afflicted children prefer to keep them at home, and this is frequently possible with help from community services. Alternatives include sheltered accommodation such as locally based hospital units (LBHUs), community homes and hostels provided by the local authority. Long-term hospital care is now discouraged, except for very severe cases or those with extreme "challenging behaviour", but people with learning disability and superadded psychiatric or behavioural disorders may well require acute admission to specialist units from time to time.

Children with mild learning disability are placed in ordinary schools if possible. Special schools exist for severe cases. Further training after school-leaving age is provided in Adult Training Centres. Some patients can hold ordinary jobs, others are employed in sheltered workshops.

PROGNOSIS

Mild cases have a good prognosis and are usually capable of living independently in adulthood. Some are "late developers" who eventually achieve an IQ within the normal range.

Life expectancy for severe cases used to be short, but many now survive into middle or old age.

PREVENTION

Many cases of learning disability could be prevented by:

- *Improved antenatal and obstetric care*, for example rubella immunisation for girls, treatment of Rhesus incompatibility, special care of low birthweight babies.
- *Screening of neonates*, to detect such metabolic conditions as phenylketonuria and hypothyroidism.
- *Improved infant welfare*, including immunisation programmes, early detection of mild learning disability and of impaired sight and hearing.
- *Genetic counselling*, which has become more important with recent advances in molecular genetics. For parents who have already produced a child with a gene or chromosome abnormality, it may be possible to calculate a precise risk of any future children being affected. In the case of recessive conditions, the carrier state in relatives can be determined. Genetic counselling should preferably be carried out as a planned procedure, rather than delayed until a new pregnancy is already in progress.
- *Prenatal diagnosis*: many congenital abnormalities can now be detected at an early stage of pregnancy, allowing the option of aborting an affected foetus should the mother choose this course. Techniques include:
    - *ultrasound*: offered to pregnant women at 16–18 weeks to confirm gestational age and detect major structural abnormalities
    - *serum alpha-fetoprotein* (AFP): also offered at 16–18 weeks. Raised levels suggest a neural tube defect such as anencephaly or myelomeningocele. Low levels suggest Down's syndrome
    - *amniocentesis*: offered at 16–18 weeks if AFP is abnormal. Amniotic fluid is sampled by the transabdominal route. Foetal chromosomes are examined, and specific genetic defects excluded using enzyme estimations or gene probes. Amniocentesis carries a small risk of causing miscarriage, infection, or damage to the child
    - *chorionic villus biopsy* (CVB): offered at 6–8 weeks for high-risk pregnancies only. Chromosome and gene abnormalities can

be detected. Chorion sampling is carried out by the trans-vaginal or transabdominal route, and carries a small risk of causing miscarriage.

Before such tests are carried out, the mother (and father) should be informed about their purpose, their accuracy, the implications of both positive and negative results, and any risks attached to them.

Some important specific causes of learning disability will be described in the text. The following box gives a fuller list, but is not complete; new genetic syndromes are continually being identified.

SOME SPECIFIC CAUSES OF LEARNING DISABILITY

Autosomal Chromosome Abnormalities:
  Down's syndrome*
  Trisomy D (Trisomy 13; Patau's syndrome)
  Trisomy E (Trisomy 18; Edwards' syndrome)
  "Cri du chat" syndrome

Sex Chromosome Abnormalities:
  Males:
    Fragile X syndrome (Martin–Bell)*
    XYY syndrome*
    XXY syndrome (Klinefelter's)*

  Females:
    XO syndrome (Turner's)*
    XXX syndrome*

Autosomal Dominant Gene Abnormalities:
  Tuberous sclerosis*

Autosomal Recessive Gene Abnormalities
  Phenylketonuria*
  Homocystinuria – an aminoaciduria
  Hartnup disease – an aminoaciduria
  Maple syrup urine disease – an aminoaciduria
  Galactosaemia*
  Tay–Sachs' disease*
  Gaucher's syndrome – lipid storage disorder
  Niemann–Pick disease – lipid storage disorder

continues

— *continued* —

Hand–Schueller–Christian disease – lipid storage disorder
Hurler's syndrome (Gargoylism) – mucopolysaccharide storage disorder
Laurence–Moon–Biedl syndrome*
Congenital hypothyroidism*

Sex-linked Recessive Gene Abnormalities
Lesch–Nyhan syndrome*
Hunter's syndrome – mucopolysaccharide storage disorder

Prenatal Infection
Cytomegalovirus*
Toxoplasmosis*
Rubella*
Syphilis*

Birth Complications
Birth injury*
Rhesus incompatibility*

Postnatal damage
Encephalitis, meningitis
HIV infection
Severe head injury
Lead poisoning*

Miscellaneous
Hydrocephalus*
Microcephaly*

*See following text.

CHROMOSOMAL ABNORMALITIES

Abnormalities of the autosomal chromosomes usually cause severe learning disability combined with widespread anatomical deformities, but the effect of sex chromosome abnormalities is more variable.

Autosomal Chromosomes

Down's syndrome is caused by one of two conditions, trisomy 21 or translocation of chromosome 21. It is the most common specific cause of learning disability, occurring in 1 per 650 pregnancies.

Trisomy 21 does not run in families, but becomes more frequent with increasing maternal age:

Maternal Age	Frequency of Trisomy 21 [per 1000 births]
under 35	1
35–39	4
40–44	13
over 45	35

Translocation of chromosome 21, which is not related to maternal age, may result from mosaicism in either parent in which case there is a likelihood of future pregnancies also being affected. In other cases it occurs sporadically.

Learning disability, often severe, is always present. Physical features include a typical facial appearance with slanting palpebral fissures, short little finger with only one palmar crease ("trident hand" and "simian crease"), hypotonic muscles, cardiac defects (10% of patients), and high susceptibility to chest infections, lymphatic leukaemia, and premature ageing. Patients used to die young but many now live till middle or old age, often developing Alzheimer's disease (Ch 10) in their 40s; an observation which helped to locate an Alzheimer's gene to chromosome 21.

There are differing opinions as to whether all pregnant women should be offered antenatal screening for detection of Down's syndrome; certainly older mothers, and those with a previously affected baby, should have the option to be screened.

Sex Chromosomes

Sex chromosome abnormalities are described here although they are not always associated with learning disability.

Male Phenotype

Fragile X (*Martin–Bell syndrome*) is the next most common genetic cause of learning disability after Down's syndrome. The long arm of the X chromosome appears to have a fragile tip when grown in special media, due to a gene with multiple abnormal DNA triplicate repeat sequences (of CGG). Fragile X syndrome is a common cause of severe learning disability in males, and causes lesser degrees of disability in some carrier females. Affected males have large testes (macroorchidism), "bat ears" and long faces. Psychotic symptoms, aggressive or socially impaired behaviour associated with social anxiety, and language impairments are common. Screening in pregnancy for women from affected families offers the possibility of aborting foetuses with Fragile X.

XYY syndrome is associated with low IQ, infertility, neurological disorders, tallness, skeletal disorders and myopia, but some cases are phenotypically normal.

XXY syndrome (*Klinefelter's syndrome*) comprises hypogonadism, infertility, tallness, effeminate body shape and usually a low IQ. Testosterone therapy may render the appearance more masculine.

Female Phenotype

XO syndrome (*Turner's syndrome*) comprises ovarian dysgenesis, short stature, webbed neck and sometimes coarctation of the aorta. IQ may be normal or low, and visuospatial disorders are often present. Patients are infertile, but oestrogen therapy may render their appearance more feminine.

XXX syndrome (*triple X, "superfemale"*) is sometimes associated with low IQ and physical abnormalities, but other cases are phenotypically normal. Patients are not infertile, but their children may have various chromosome abnormalities. Women with more than three X chromosomes have learning disability and numerous physical defects.

GENE ABNORMALITIES

Autosomal Dominant

Tuberous sclerosis is characterised by learning disability (in about 40% of cases), epilepsy (in about 60% of cases) and facial angiofibromas. Nodules of neuroglia, sometimes calcified, occur in the brain and show on a brain scan. Muscular and vascular tumours may occur in various organs, and "cafe au lait spots" and "shagreen patches" on the skin. Disease-determining gene loci have been found on chromosomes 9 and 16.

Autosomal Recessive

Phenylketonuria occurs in 4 per 100 000 live births. It results from a defect in phenylalanine hydroxylase, the enzyme which converts phenylalanine to tyrosine, or from enzyme defects in the subsequent metabolic pathway. Phenylpyruvic acid and other abnormal metabolites of phenylalanine are present in the urine after three weeks of age, enabling a screening test to be carried out. Carriers of the gene can be detected by a phenylalanine loading test for genetic counselling purposes. Patients have fair colouring, because melanin production is impaired. Untreated cases have severe learning disability, but if a low phenylalanine diet is started in infancy and continued until age ten, intellectual development may approach normal.

Galactosaemia results from a defect of galactose 1-phosphate uridyltransferase, the enzyme which converts galactose to glucose. Vomiting, jaundice and hepatosplenomegaly are present from infancy, and cataracts develop later. It can be detected by finding galactose in the urine. A diet free from milk and other galactose-containing foods ameliorates the symptoms.

Tay–Sachs' disease is a degenerative condition of the central nervous system due to an abnormality of lipid metabolism. It occurs mostly in Jewish families. A cherry-red spot appears on the macula after a few months of age and is followed by optic atrophy and blindness. Epileptic fits develop, and patients usually die about the age of two years.

Hurler's syndrome (*gargoylism*) is a disorder of the metabolism of mucopolysaccharides, which accumulate in the brain and other organs, causing hepatosplenomegaly. Aggressive temperament may be associated.

Laurence–Moon–Biedl syndrome comprises learning disability, retinitis pigmentosa, polydactyly, obesity and hypogonadism.

Congenital hypothyroidism, due to deficiency of one of the enzymes involved in thyroxine synthesis, causes general retardation of development with lethargy and a puffy appearance. Symptoms can be alleviated by lifelong thyroxine replacement therapy.

Sex-linked Recessive

Lesch–Nyhan syndrome results from a defect of purine metabolism, with accumulation of uric acid. There is severe learning disability, self-mutilation, spasticity and choreo-athetosis. 5-Hydroxytryptophan treatment may ameliorate the behaviour disorder.

ACQUIRED HANDICAP

Prenatal Infections

Cytomegalovirus is the commonest form of intrauterine infection to cause learning disability. The mother is usually symptom-free. The child has microcephaly, necrotising haemorrhaging encephalitis and intracerebral calcification, and may die in early life.

Toxoplasmosis is a protozoal infection which causes learning disability, choroidoretinitis and miliary intracranial calcification. Maternal infection can be detected by serological testing in pregnancy.

Rubella, if contracted by a woman during the first trimester of pregnancy, can cause learning disability, deafness, cataract and cardiac lesions in the child. Such cases are preventable by vaccination of those girls who have not developed natural immunity to rubella in childhood.

Congenital syphilis, now rare, causes learning disability, deafness, keratitis, and malformed teeth, and general paralysis of the insane (GPI) develops in adolescence. Serological tests may be negative. It can be prevented by screening of pregnant women with antisyphilitic treatment for them if required.

Birth Complications

Birth injury, or rhesus incompatibility, may cause learning disability associated with either spasticity or athetoid movements of one or more limbs (cerebral palsy).

Postnatal Damage

Lead poisoning may result from exposure to high concentrations of petrol fumes, or from sucking lead-painted objects, which children already handicapped by low IQ or sensory impairments are particularly likely to do. It causes mild intellectual impairment, anaemia with basophil stippling of red cells, and a "lead line" on the gums and epiphyses.

MISCELLANEOUS

Hydrocephalus has various causes: congenital malformation of the fourth ventricle associated with spina bifida, meningitis or a brainstem tumour in childhood, or rarely a sex-linked inherited condition. Insertion of a shunt ameliorates brain damage.

Microcephaly may result from a recessive autosomal gene and comprises severe learning disability, overactivity, and a low cephalic index which gives a bird-like appearance. Microcephaly may also result from other causes such as radiation or cytomegalovirus infection in utero.

FURTHER READING

Bernal J, Hollins S (1995) Psychiatric illness and learning disability; a dual diagnosis. *Advances in Psychiatric Treatment* **1**: 138–145

Reid AH (1994) Psychiatry and learning disability. *British Journal of Psychiatry* **164**: 613–618

Thapar A, Gottesman II, Owen MJ, O'Donovan MC, McGuffin P (1994) The genetics of mental retardation. *British Journal of Psychiatry* **164**: 747–758

Turk J (1992) The fragile-X syndrome. On the way to a behavioural phenotype. *British Journal of Psychiatry* **160**: 24–35

20

Psychiatry of Old Age

The psychiatry of old age is of growing importance, because the proportion of elderly people in the UK population is increasing. "Old age" services as opposed to "general adult" services may take patients over the age of 65, or 75, depending on local arrangements.

Psychiatric illness becomes more common with advancing age. This is because elderly people have a high prevalence of cerebral and systemic diseases which can cause organic brain syndromes, and because they are often subject to emotional stresses and loss. These include the deaths of spouse, siblings and friends; loss of occupation, company and income following retirement; deterioration in bodily functions; the prospect of further ageing and death; and sometimes, both within private households and institutions, mistreatment by those with the responsibility for care ("elder abuse").

FREQUENCY

Community surveys show the following approximate prevalence figures for psychiatric illness in people over the age of 65:

Depression	15%
Anxiety and phobias	15%
Dementia	10%

Prevalence rises sharply after about the age of 75.

CLINICAL SYNDROMES

Depression (Ch 5) is the most common psychiatric disorder in old people, and first admission rates for depression are highest in the 50–70 age group. Mixed anxiety-depressive states frequently present in primary care with psychiatric symptoms, insomnia, physical problems or social difficulties ("failure to cope").

Most depressive episodes recover in the short term, but long-term prognosis is worse than for younger patients. At least 70% develop further episodes.

Suicide rates rise with age, and suicide in elderly people is often associated with clinical depression as well as with social isolation.

Depression in old people may be associated with cognitive impairment and therefore be difficult to distinguish from early dementia. A careful history, mental state examination, and a brain scan often help to make the distinction, but the two disorders may co-exist.

Antidepressant drugs are effective but low doses should initially be used because unwanted effects, for example postural hypotension with tricyclics, are more severe than in younger adults. If successful, antidepressants should be continued for 1–2 years in old people, perhaps even for life, because of the high likelihood of relapse. ECT is readily considered in the elderly, as it acts more quickly than medication and, apart from transient mental confusion, often has fewer unwanted effects. ECT may be lifesaving in a severely depressed patient who is dehydrated due to refusal to eat and drink.

Mania (Ch 5): although first admission rates for mania show a slight increase with age, it remains an unusual presentation. It is important to exclude physical causes such as a brain tumour, cerebrovascular disease, or medication such as steroids, especially if a careful search (old casenotes, interviewing relatives) fails to reveal any previous history. Patients with longstanding bipolar illness tend to suffer less mania and more depression if they survive into old age. Transient depressive symptoms occur during most manic illnesses in the elderly. Physical illness or injuries often result from self-neglect and over-activity, so inpatient treatment is desirable.

Schizophrenia (Ch 4) and *Paranoid Disorders* (Ch 8): about 14% of schizophrenic illnesses in women, and 4% in men, start after the age of 65 and almost always take the paranoid form with good preservation of general personality. It is important to check for deafness or blindness which may be treatable. Social activity, for example through a day centre or residential home, may be helpful if the patient will accept it. Antipsychotic drugs are used but results are sometimes disappointing.

Case Example

A widower aged 73 had lived an increasingly isolated life since retirement. His GP was called to see him as an emergency by the police, to whom he had made frequent 999 calls alleging that his neighbours were trying to murder him with gas. Apart from his obvious delusions, the man was otherwise in good health. He did not believe that he was in any way unwell, and was compulsorily admitted, after a domiciliary visit from the duty psychiatrist, to a psychiatric ward under the Mental Health Act 1983. He was unwilling to take oral medication, but his symptoms partially resolved with a small dose of a depot antipsychotic injection. Although he was able to be discharged, he remained isolated and generally suspicious, and his community psychiatric nurse (CPN) frequently had difficulty in persuading him to have his injection.

Neurotic disorders (Ch 6): reactions to bereavement or other stressors may produce brief adjustment disorders in the elderly, just as in younger people, however it is unusual for a prolonged neurotic condition to become established in an elderly person who has previously been free of such symptoms. Indeed, most people suffering from neuroses are said to get better rather than worse as they grow older. Such a first presentation in an elderly person should raise suspicion of organic disorder or depressive illness.

Dementia, delirium and other organic brain syndromes: see Ch 10.

Case Example

A woman of 83 had been diagnosed as suffering from moderate to severe dementia of Alzheimer's type, but was able to remain at home because of the devoted care of her 62-year-old daughter.

continues

┌───┐

─────continued─────

Her behaviour became much more agitated and confused over a period of two days, alternating with periods of drowsiness; her urine had become foul-smelling over this time. The GP and CPN diagnosed acute-on-chronic confusion due to urinary tract infection, and continued to look after the patient at home, for her daughter wished to avoid hospital admission. With antibiotics, a change of catheter and a course of the sedative major tranquilliser thioridazine, the patient's condition returned to normal over a few days. Her daughter nevertheless appeared exhausted, and regular respite care admissions were arranged to ease her burden.

└───┘

Alcohol and Drugs: alcohol misuse (Ch 13) may become a problem in old age, but is often concealed. Depression, loneliness and boredom, perhaps following the death of a spouse, are common precipitants. Drug misuse (Ch 12) usually involves prescribed drugs, such as benzodiazepines which often cause ataxia and cognitive impairment in this age group. If an elderly person with unrecognised alcohol or drug dependence develops an intercurrent illness and/or is admitted to hospital, withdrawal symptoms may ensue.

ASSESSMENT

Although it is important to reach a psychiatric and/or medical diagnosis, identification of the practical problems facing the patient may be the most urgent requirement. Often the point at issue is whether he or she is able to cope at home. This may hinge on something as mundane as, for example, whether a neighbour who does the shopping is prepared to continue doing so.

An assessment in the patient's home surroundings is more meaningful than one carried out in hospital, and an interview with an informant is highly desirable especially if there is any question of cognitive impairment. The timespan of the illness can be crucial in making a diagnosis; a mental illness such as depression will usually come on over weeks, a dementia over months, and an acute confusional state over hours or days.

Psychiatric history and mental state are recorded in the usual way (Ch 3). Particular emphasis should be placed on medical factors and social circumstances, and it is essential to test cognitive function. Physical examination may well reveal undiagnosed pathology which needs attention.

Standardised instruments for interviewing elderly patients include the CAMDEX (Cambridge Examination for Mental Disorders of the Elderly) and GMSS (Geriatric Mental State Schedule). Short questionnaires for assessing cognitive function include the Mini Mental State (MMS) and Abbreviated Mental Test Score (AMTS).

SPECIFIC TREATMENTS

Psychotropic drugs (Ch 23) should be used in small starting doses because:

- metabolism and excretion are slow
- both therapeutic effects and unwanted effects may be found with low doses
- medical conditions necessitating caution in drug use may be present
- interactions with other medication may occur.

Forgetfulness and other factors may lead to poor compliance, so single-drug therapy in once-daily dosage is desirable.

The prescriber should become familiar with a small number of preparations and their unwanted effects, make a special effort to gain the trust of the patient, and pay great attention to explanation and detail. For example, someone with severe arthritis of the hands may not be able to take tablets which are dispensed in a "blister pack"; and a change in colour of tablet, or from tablet to capsule, may be worrying for an elderly person.

Antidepressants: either *tricyclics* or *SSRIs* may be used. Tricyclics are cheaper, have predictable unwanted effects, and can be started at very low doses. Some authorities recommend drugs of secondary tricyclic structure, such as *nortriptyline*, because anticholinergic and hypotensive effects are less than with tertiary tricyclics such as amitriptyline. The major advantage of the SSRIs is their lack of toxicity in overdosage. *Lithium* is used in prophylaxis of depression and mania.

Sedatives for use in psychosis or agitation include:

- *promazine*, an effective sedative but weak antipsychotic
- *haloperidol*, often effective in doses as low as 1 mg, but having marked Parkinsonian side-effects
- *thioridazine*, a good non-Parkinsonian antipsychotic, but may induce confusion because of its anticholinergic properties.

Hypnotics and "minor" tranquillisers were overprescribed in the past, creating a large population of elderly long-term users. However, it is possible that the pendulum has swung too far against these drugs; provided they are used judiciously in line with *British National Formulary* recommendations, they remain a safe and effective treatment for transient neurotic states such as insomnia after a bereavement.

ECT (Ch 24) may be used if the patient is fit for anaesthetic, and is often better tolerated than antidepressant drugs, but many patients need long-term drug prophylaxis also.

Psychological treatments (Ch 22): psychotherapy in its briefer forms may be helpful. Intensive exploratory work is inappropriate because major changes in personality or attitudes are not likely to be achieved. Individual or group treatment may be focused on adaptation to bereavement or the other losses of old age. *Marital therapy* may be indicated, because conflicts in a marriage often become more obvious when the partners are brought into continuous contact by retirement or restricted mobility. Special techniques for this age group include *reality orientation* (RO) and *reminiscence therapy*. *Behaviour therapy techniques*, including practical memory aids, may be of benefit for demented patients.

ORGANISATION OF SERVICES

The vast bulk of psychiatric disorders are coped with by patients themselves, their relatives and carers; some cases are recognised and treated in primary care, but only the minority reach secondary care. General practitioners have sometimes been criticised for not knowing about such problems in patients on their list, but there is evidence that GPs avoid making these diagnoses if they feel, as is often unfortunately the case, that local psychiatric services for the elderly are overstretched.

Multidisciplinary teams in old age psychiatry, as in general adult psychiatry (Ch 26), include doctors, nurses, psychologists, social workers and occupational therapists. They work in liaison with primary health care teams, social services, and gerontology departments.

Many of the problems identified in a comprehensive assessment are *social* rather than psychiatric, and require practical interventions accordingly. For example, a depressed patient who is living alone in poor accommodation will be unlikely to make a good recovery with antidepressant medication alone. Attending a day centre might combat loneliness and improve nutrition, and a social worker would advise about housing and social security benefits.

Physical problems also need to be addressed. Undiagnosed medical illness, inappropriate medication, and dietary deficiencies are common in this age-group.

Hospital admission is frequently valuable to treat illness or, commonly, to relieve a social crisis. However, hospitalisation should not be undertaken too lightly. Many old people survive in their own homes through a complex network of informal care and company from relatives, friends, church, the voluntary sector and domestic pets, and this network may prove impossible to reassemble following an admission. If the patient does go into hospital, a gradual discharge with increasing periods of home leave is the rule.

Inpatient facilities include assessment wards for functional psychiatric illness and for demented patients. These are separate from the wards for younger adults, but some facilities may be shared with physicians for the elderly.

Respite admissions at regular planned intervals are particularly valued by relatives, and provide patients themselves with care and company, and an opportunity for thorough medical and nursing review.

Day hospital care is often preferable to inpatient admission, and also less costly.

Home care: a "package" of "community care" can not only support people with continuing difficulties, but can also be used as a treatment, with increased support at times of crisis.

Recent legislation has encouraged care in the community, as institutional beds have closed, but the changes have not been properly resourced and old age psychiatry remains a "Cinderella" speciality with many unmet needs; it is clear that the health and social services would be entirely unable to cope were it not for unpaid carers and the voluntary sector.

A major change has been the new responsibility of local authority social services to "purchase" appropriate care for individuals. This care may range from provision of home helps, laundry and meals-on-wheels, to residential accommodation. Such measures can no longer be directly prescribed by health services, so good local day-to-day working relationships with social workers are vital.

Long-term institutional care is desirable for some patients, but the number of hospital beds for this purpose has been greatly decreased in recent years. Alternatives include warden-controlled housing or residential homes run by local authorities, or privately run rest homes and nursing homes.

FURTHER READING

Books

Jacoby R, Oppenheimer C (1991) *Psychiatry in the Elderly*. Oxford University Press: Oxford
Pitt B, Naguib M (1995) *Seminars in Psychiatry for the Elderly*. Gaskell Books: London

Review Articles

Burns A, Baldwin R (1994) Prescribing psychotropic drugs for the elderly. *Advances in Psychiatric Treatment* **1**: 23–31

21

Forensic Psychiatry

Forensic psychiatrists are general adult psychiatrists with special knowledge of offending behaviour among the mentally ill, and the law relating to this. Their role includes:

- Work in prisons.
- Running Medium Secure Units and Special Hospitals.
- Supervision of outpatients.
- Consultation service to general psychiatrists.
- Psychiatric reports for courts/lawyers.
- Court Diversion Schemes for mentally disordered offenders (MDOs).

Considerable political and media interest in forensic psychiatry has followed a recent succession of well-publicised individual "scandals"; for example, suicides in prison leading to calls to remove MDOs from the criminal justice system, and crimes by MDOs leading to calls for them to be detained permanently in psychiatric hospitals. Measures such as the Supervision Register and Care Programme Approach (Ch 26) have been introduced, in part, in response to such pressures.

OFFENDING BEHAVIOUR

Community surveys show that offending behaviour is extremely common, and that the vast majority of the population have broken the law in some way at some time. Generally speaking, offending behaviour is commoner in males, and peaks during the teenage years, gradually becoming less frequent thereafter. Most cases involve minor property offences such as theft and vandalism. Only a tiny proportion are reported, and only a fraction of these result in conviction. Of people convicted, the proportion going on to become persistent serious offenders is small.

Causes of offending behaviour are predominantly social and environmental, rather than psychiatric. Juvenile delinquency (Ch 18) often persists into adulthood as criminality and/or antisocial personality. Criminality tends to run in families. Twin and adoption studies indicate some specific genetic component to this inheritance, but other factors such as coming from a large impoverished family, poor parenting, a culture of criminal behaviour in the neighbourhood and school, and low intelligence are thought to be of greater influence.

Male offenders outnumber female ones about 10-fold, and male prisoners outnumber female ones about 30-fold. Both cultural and biological factors contribute to this discrepancy. Female prisoners have more mental and physical disease than male ones.

PREDICTING VIOLENCE AND DANGEROUSNESS

"Risk assessment" is an important part of the work of forensic and other psychiatrists. Dangerousness varies according to the situation, and is impossible to predict accurately. Risk factors include:

- Past history of violence: this is by far the most important guide to present and future risk.
- Personal/family history of criminality/substance misuse/suicidal behaviour.
- Preoccupation with, or threats of, violence.
- Psychiatric disorder, especially with paranoid delusions.
- Cold/callous explosive/antisocial personality traits.
- Impulsivity/irritability/emotional arousal.
- Ready availability of a weapon and a victim.

In a potentially violent situation in psychiatric practice, consider the above factors with due regard for intuition and common sense. If the interviewer feels anxiety or fear, it is prudent to adjourn the interview to seek assistance and advice.

FACILITIES FOR MENTALLY DISORDERED OFFENDERS

Special Hospitals

Special Hospitals exist for treatment of patients with mental disorder, mainly psychosis, sociopathy or learning disability, who have committed violent crimes. They comprise Broadmoor, Rampton and Ashworth in England, and Carstairs in Scotland. All patients are compulsorily admitted and detained under the Mental Health Act 1983, the majority from the courts, some from prisons or psychiatric hospitals. Violence to others, sex offences and arson are frequent reasons for admission. Prospective admissions are assessed by Special Hospital staff, the main criteria being the presence of mental disorder and a "grave and immediate" risk to others. Most patients stay several years but about 50% eventually become fit for transfer to a local psychiatric unit in preparation for discharge to the community.

Regional Secure Units

Regional Secure Units (RSUs) have been set up around the country, in line with current policy to expand the number of "medium secure" beds in each health district, so that the majority of psychiatric patients with violent behaviour, and of psychiatrically disturbed offenders, can receive treatment locally and only the most dangerous ones be sent to Special Hospitals.

A typical RSU might have twenty beds, under the supervision of a consultant forensic psychiatrist and associated multidisciplinary team. Inpatient beds are frequently full, as referrals of "difficult to manage" (not necessarily forensic) patients from general psychiatric services are increasing. Such patients would formerly have been contained in traditional mental hospitals, but violence or threats of violence often cannot be adequately managed in DGH units or by community care (Ch 26).

Prison Medical Services

Just as most mental disorder in the community as a whole is managed in primary care, so most mental disorder among prisoners is managed by the Prison Medical Service. Most prisons also have regular sessional commitments from a visiting general adult psychiatrist or forensic psychiatrist, who will advise on diagnosis and management, either in the general wings or the prison hospital. Compulsory treatment under the Mental Health Act 1983 (Ch 27) is not, however, permitted in prisons. Sometimes it is necessary to transfer an inmate to psychiatric hospital, not necessarily under conditions of security, and the psychiatrist is able to assist in placement.

Surveys of male prisoners indicate that about 30% can be diagnosed as having a mental abnormality. Sociopathy and alcoholism are the main diagnoses but learning disability, functional psychosis, organic brain disease and epilepsy are also found in excess. In some cases this disorder has not been recognised. Others are in prison because no psychiatric hospital place can be found for them. However the presence of certain psychiatric disorders, for example personality disorder/substance misuse/treated chronic mental illness, does not necessarily mean that prison is an inappropriate placement.

Diversion Schemes

In some Magistrates' Courts, regular attendance by psychiatrists or other trained staff allows psychiatrically disturbed persons coming before the Court to be diverted as appropriate from the criminal justice system into the health care system.

Diversion also happens at an even earlier stage, for example the custody sergeant at a police station may ask the police surgeon to examine an arrested person and, if a mental disorder is present, the help of local psychiatric services is sought.

Social and Probation Services

These services have a close relationship with forensic psychiatry, including:

- Social and probation reports on offenders before the court.
- Resettlement of offenders.
- Probation and bail hostels.

For example, a mentally disordered person convicted of a crime may be put on probation, with psychiatric treatment as a condition of this.

Failure to cooperate with treatment would be a breach of the probation order and result in the offender being brought back before the court.

Primary Care

Many offenders, especially released prisoners, are not registered with a GP. This situation often adds to the difficulties of providing adequate medical care for this population, with its high rate of both physical and psychiatric illness. The special community clinics for homeless people which have been set up in some cities may help to meet these needs.

TREATMENT: GENERAL CONSIDERATIONS

If a clearly identified mental illness appears directly related to the offending behaviour, the prognosis can be very good. For example, a man with schizophrenia who smashes up a television shop because he believes it is transmitting harmful rays will be unlikely to repeat this behaviour if his delusions resolve with treatment.

In other cases, mental disorder may co-exist with offending behaviour without being a significant causative factor, so that treatment of the disorder has little impact on the behaviour.

Substance misuse is very common among offenders. If, for example, a chronic alcoholic can be rehabilitated, he will be less likely to commit drunkenness and public order offences. Many prisons run AA groups for this reason. However, it is not always appropriate to remove a person from the criminal justice system on the grounds of substance misuse alone. Motivation to stop substance misuse may appear higher before an impending court appearance than later proves to be the case.

Psychological or behavioural treatments have been tried, irrespective of the presence of mental disorder, for a variety of habitual offenders, for example those convicted of car theft, "road rage" and assault. Few if any of these treatments have been shown to be effective in randomised controlled trials, and they tend to be regarded cautiously by psychiatrists. If they are to be provided, prison psychology services, probation or social services are the best source.

PSYCHIATRIC COURT REPORTS

Court reports should be written in non-technical language, as they will be used by lawyers and other lay persons. Two sides of A4 are ample for most cases. Before beginning work, the wise psychiatrist obtains the written agreement of the person requesting the report to pay a fee, as this work is not part of NHS practice. Reports are most frequently requested by courts, in which case the psychiatrist will often work with the probation officer, and by defence lawyers. It is crucial to establish clearly the question behind the request, for example is the court asking about fitness to plead or advice about sentencing?

The following scheme is appropriate:

- Name, age, address, occupation, marital status.
- Sources of information: when and where the psychiatrist interviewed the defendant, other informants interviewed and documents consulted.
- Index offence.
- Forensic history.
- Medical and psychiatric history, including history of present illness (if any).
- Personal background, including family history.
- Present social circumstances.
- Substance use.
- Circumstances of index offence, including opinion on mental state at the time of offending.
- Present mental state.
- Opinion, including advice on specific points raised by the person requesting the report.

Case Example

An unemployed man aged 38 presented himself to Casualty with the complaint of "hearing voices". He admitted to recent drug use, and the likely diagnosis seemed drug-induced psychosis. He was admitted to a psychiatric ward informally, and rapidly improved with oral antipsychotic medication, but discharged himself before a full assessment had been made. He did not attend follow-up, but presented again with similar symptoms shortly afterwards. On this

continues

——*continued*——

occasion no beds were available and he was sent home with medication. Two weeks later, his consultant was surprised to receive a request from the local Magistrates' Court for a psychiatric report "to assist in sentencing for a number of motoring offences".

It emerged after obtaining old notes that this man had been brought up in a large and chaotic family, of long-standing criminal tendencies, and had been subject to a mixture of neglect and abuse. He had spent his life taking, selling, repairing and even living in cars, and had multiple convictions for vehicle offences; none of a variety of sentences had influenced this behaviour. His only psychiatric history was the complaint of hearing voices during his last term of imprisonment; he had been transferred to hospital, only to abscond shortly afterwards. His probation officer indicated to the psychiatrist that the Court was very keen for him to be taken on for medical treatment, as they felt that other disposals would be ineffective.

At interview, residual psychotic symptoms were still apparent, but resolving. The man was frank about his drug use, and also about his intentions to continue with his offending behaviour.

The psychiatrist's report indicated that his personality appeared to have been damaged by his unsatisfactory upbringing, but that no treatable mental illness was present; that his psychotic symptoms appeared due to a combination of illegal drug use and the stress of actual or impending imprisonment; and made no recommendations to the court as to disposal.

In the event, he was given a six-month prison sentence during which he developed recurrent psychotic symptoms which were well contained with antipsychotic medication. He was released as soon as possible under remission rules, did not attend a psychiatric follow-up appointment, and continued to offend.

PSYCHIATRIC ASPECTS OF SPECIFIC OFFENCES

Homicide

"Unlawful homicide" includes *murder*, *manslaughter* and *infanticide*. The legal definition of murder requires that the crime was premeditated and the accused was fully responsible for the act. If these conditions are not fulfilled, the offence becomes manslaughter.

Infanticide is a defence when a child less than a year old is killed by its mother, who is "suffering from a mental imbalance attributable to the effects of giving birth or to the consequent lactation".

There are 400–500 homicides per year in England and Wales. In about 75% of cases, killer and victim are well known to each other. About 50% of killers have a serious psychiatric disorder and about 15% commit suicide soon after their crime.

The main disorders which can lead to homicide are:

- *Psychoses, usually with delusions*: depressed people may kill their children or other close relatives because of a delusion that they are going to suffer an even worse fate. Schizophrenia may lead to homicide through paranoid delusions. Puerperal psychosis accounts for some, but not all, cases of infanticide.
- *Sociopathic personality disorder.*
- *Drug-induced states.*
- *Morbid jealousy.*
- *Learning disability*, in which frustration may be expressed by violence.
- *Epileptic automatism*: this is rare.
- *Automatism during sleep*: individuals prone to sleepwalking or night terrors occasionally kill during sleep. This rare defence is hard to prove.
- *Organic brain disease.*

The presence of a mental disorder may permit a murder charge to be reduced to manslaughter on the grounds of *diminished responsibility*, under the Homicide Act 1957. A verdict of murder always carries a sentence of life imprisonment, but manslaughter may receive any sentence, including a hospital order under the Mental Health Act 1983, or discharge.

Less often, a mentally abnormal offender accused of murder or other serious crime is found *"unfit to plead"* and sent directly to a psychiatric hospital, sometimes being required to stand trial later on if the psychiatric condition improves. The grounds for being unfit to plead are inability to: instruct counsel, appreciate the significance of pleading, challenge a juror, examine a witness, or understand the evidence or court procedure.

A rare plea, in practice reserved for murder cases, is *"not guilty by reason of insanity"* when the offender fulfils the MacNaughten Rules, that is he either did not know the nature and quality of his act, or did not know that it was wrong. A deluded patient is assumed to be under the same degree of responsibility as if the delusions were true. If this plea is successful, the accused is sent to a psychiatric hospital.

About half of those accused of murder claim amnesia for the event, but this is not an adequate defence, nor is voluntary intoxication with alcohol or drugs. Automatism, in epileptics or sleepwalkers, does make an acceptable defence.

A child under 10 cannot be accused of murder.

Rape

Rape is sexual intercourse with a person who does not consent. Many cases are probably not reported to the police. Most rape victims are women, but male rape is an increasingly recognised problem. The following types of rapist are described:

- *Inhibited* men who are unable to form normal sexual relationships.
- *Aggressive* violent men with contempt for women.
- *Sadistic* men who commit premeditated rapes.
- Men with *psychiatric illness* or *learning disability*.
- *Group rape*, by gangs of youths whose members would probably not commit the crime individually.
- *"Date rape"*, recently much publicised, in which a man claims that a woman consented to have sex with him, but she denies this.

Of convicted rapists, 90% do not repeat their crime, but the aggressive and sadistic types often do so, and therefore may require long-term secure detention.

Psychological therapies and/or antilibidinal drugs may be used in the management of rapists. Victims of rape may develop psychiatric disorders, such as post-traumatic stress disorder or sexual dysfunction, and early counselling may help prevent these after-effects.

Arson

About 40% of serious fires are started deliberately. Types of arsonist include:

- *Criminally motivated*, for example obtaining insurance money or concealing evidence of another crime.
- *Psychotic* patients motivated by delusions.

- Those with *sociopathic personality* and/or *low intelligence* who start fires for excitement, sexual stimulation or revenge. They often repeat the offence and require secure detention.

Shoplifting

The law does not distinguish shoplifting (theft from shops) from other kinds of theft, but it has been studied separately by psychiatrists. It is predominantly a crime of women. Types include:

- Straightforward *theft*.
- Search for *excitement* by those of sociopathic personality.
- *Psychiatric disorders* including depressive illness (especially in middle-aged women), mania, schizophrenia, dementia, learning disability.
- *Absent-mindedness* due to medical conditions such as epilepsy or hypoglycaemia, or prescribed drugs such as benzodiazepines.

Other topics with forensic implications include antisocial personality (Ch 7), sexual deviations (Ch 17), juvenile delinquency (Ch 18), child abuse (Ch 18), the Mental Health Act (Ch 27).

FURTHER READING

Books

Bluglass R, Bowden P (eds) (1990) *Principles and Practice of Forensic Psychiatry*. Churchill Livingstone: Edinburgh

Chiswick D, Cope R (eds) (1995) *Seminars in Forensic Psychiatry*. Gaskell Books: London

Faulk M (1988) *Basic Forensic Psychiatry*. Blackwell: Oxford

Review Articles

Bluglass R (1995) Preparing a medico-legal report. *Advances in Psychiatric Treatment* 1: 131–137

Joseph PLA (1994) Psychiatric assessment at the magistrates court. *British Journal of Psychiatry* 164: 722–724

Vinestock MD (1966) Risk assessment. "A word to the wise"? *Advances in Psychiatric Treatment* 2: 3–10

III

Treatment

22

Psychological Treatment

The term *psychological treatment* is largely synonymous with *psychotherapy*, defined by Storr as "the art of alleviating personal difficulties through the agency of words and a personal professional relationship". Some modern psychotherapeutic techniques make use of actions, exercise, music or art as well as words. Psychotherapy may be carried out with individuals, groups, couples or families.

HISTORICAL BACKGROUND

Medicine has always recognised the importance of the patient's confiding relationship with the physician, as enshrined in the Hippocratic Oath of Ancient Greece. This non-specific psychological aspect of treatment is especially important in psychiatry. Through the years, more specific psychological approaches have been conceptualised, ranging from mediaeval notions of the "casting out of demons" in mad people to the "animal magnetism" of Mesmer in the nineteenth century.

It was only about one hundred years ago, however, that a systematic theoretical base for psychological treatment was developed in Sigmund Freud's "psychoanalysis". Although now little used in practice, psychoanalysis has been paramount in establishing the importance of psychological matters with the general public, and in providing one of the most enduringly interesting models of the mind. The work of Freud and the post-Freudians is briefly described below.

Sigmund Freud (1856–1939)

Freud's system of psychoanalysis forms the basis of modern psychodynamic psychotherapy. During psychoanalysis, in which 50-minute treatment sessions take place 3–5 times a week for several years, the patient talks about past and present events, emotions, dreams and fantasies, and uses "free association" to recall repressed or forgotten material to conscious awareness. The therapist's interpretations relate to Freud's concepts which include:

- *The model of the mind*: id (inherited, instinctive, largely unconscious, motivated by the "pleasure principle"), *ego* (largely conscious, acting according to the "reality principle" and using the ego defence mechanisms), *superego* (derived from introjection of authority figures, and equivalent to conscience).
- Stages of psychosexual development: in each of the *oral, anal, genital* and *oedipal* stages, the *libido* or sexual energy (asserted by Freud to be of prime importance in all areas of mental activity) is attached in a particular direction.
- *Transference*, in which attitudes derived from early relationships are projected onto the therapist.
- *Resistance*, in which the patient avoids exploration of a topic which is the subject of unconscious conflicts.
- *Ego defence mechanisms*: unconscious processes to reduce anxiety. include *denial, repression, rationalisation, projection, reaction formation, displacement, sublimation, intellectualisation, conversion, fixation, regression* and *introjection* (see Glossary).
- *Dreams*, in which the real or "latent" content is converted into the "manifest" content by the mental "censor" using the mechanisms of condensation, displacement and symbolism.
- *Parapraxes*: mistakes and memory lapses in everyday life which have unconscious significance.

Carl Jung (1875–1961)

Jung's system of psychotherapy, called *analytical psychology*, emphasises the exploration of dreams and the unconscious, and aims at "individuation" of the patient; this involves achieving harmony between the conscious and unconscious, and full experience of the self. Jungian concepts include:

- *Libido,* or general psychic energy, flowing between pairs of opposites such as progression–regression, conscious–unconscious, extroversion–introversion. If it is blocked in one direction pathology results, for example excess energy in the unconscious manifest as psychiatric illness.
- *The unconscious mind,* as revealed in dreams, with both personal and collective aspects, the latter including instincts, archetypes and universal symbols.
- *Personality* depends on the degree of extroversion and introversion and which of the "four functions" – thinking, feeling, sensation and intuition – is most highly developed. There is an outward personality, or "persona", and an unconscious "shadow" which has opposite characteristics.

Jung's book *Man and his Symbols* gives a readable, illustrated account of his life and work.

Melanie Klein (1882–1960)

Klein worked with children under two years old, and believed that failure of psychological development at this time was the origin of neurosis in later life. She described developmental stages: the *paranoid-schizoid position* related to the child's perception of its mother's breast first as a "good object" which is introjected, then as a "bad object" onto which aggressive feelings are projected, followed by the *depressive position* when the child becomes aware that the good and bad mother are the same and must cope with the depressive anxiety of having attacked the needed good object.

Other "neo-Freudians" include Adler, Fromm, Reich, Erikson, Sullivan, Horney, Anna Freud, Winnicot and Fairbairn.

Many of these ideas relate to the cultural, or spiritual, domains of life rather than the medical or scientific. However, many people continue to find them of great interest, and a source of validity and meaning which they may feel lacking in their everyday life.

PRINCIPLES OF PSYCHOTHERAPY TODAY

Types of Psychotherapy

The three main types in current use are:

- *Psychodynamic* (*interpretative*): exploration of early life, and re-experiencing of habitual patterns in the current relationship with the therapist, are used to explain and relieve symptoms. Modern psychodynamic methods, though based on those of Freud and the post-Freudians, use shorter and more eclectic treatment, for example brief focal therapy (Malan).
- *Behavioural*: a structured method, developed mainly by psychologists, employing practical strategies to overcome current symptoms. The principle is changing behaviour, rather than addressing presumed underlying causes or accompanying thoughts and feelings.
- *Cognitive*: based on the work of Beck, and addressing the maladaptive beliefs and attitudes presumed to contribute towards current symptoms. Cognitive therapy has become widely used in recent years.

These three approaches will be described in more detail below. Current opinion emphasises the similarities between different psychotherapies, rather than their differences, and combinations of the above techniques can be used, for example *cognitive-behavioural therapy* (see below), and *cognitive-analytical therapy* (Ryle). Many other named techniques exist, for example *interpersonal therapy* (Klerman), *client-centred therapy* (Rogers), *Gestalt therapy* (Perl), *psychodrama* (Moreno), *transactional analysis* (Berne), *hypnotherapy*, *psychosynthesis* (Assagioli): largely practised in the private sector rather than through the NHS.

Supportive psychotherapy involves discussion of problems at a simple, practical level, which may include offering advice. Any good doctor–patient relationship includes an element of supportive psychotherapy. *Counselling* was developed as a form of supportive psychotherapy to help psychiatrically normal people in difficult life situations such as bereavement or marital breakdown; the term is also used to cover more sophisticated long-term interventions having much in common with psychodynamic psychotherapy.

Psychotherapy can be usefully combined with antidepressants, or other psychotropic drugs, for patients with formal psychiatric illness.

Many psychotherapists prefer to speak of "clients" rather than "patients", however the term "patient" is retained here for the sake of consistency with the rest of the book.

Indications for Psychotherapy

The patients who respond best are those suffering from neurotic symptoms or mild personality disorders who are well motivated to change, firmly committed to treatment, able to understand psychological concepts, prepared to take responsibility for decisions, reasonably intelligent and verbally fluent. Critics might say that patients fulfilling all these criteria are not in pressing need of therapy. Contrary to previous belief, older patients can benefit as well as younger ones.

Contraindications for Psychotherapy

Patients who have psychotic illnesses, are taking large quantities of drugs (prescribed or illicit) or alcohol, or have severe personality disorders are usually considered unsuitable.

Unwanted Effects of Psychotherapy

- *Excessive dependence* on therapy or the therapist.
- *Intensive techniques may cause distress* and, occasionally, precipitate acute psychiatric breakdown.
- *Disorders for which physical treatments are required*, for example severe depression, or medical illness presenting with psychological symptoms, may be missed, especially by non-medical therapists.
- *Ineffective psychotherapy wastes time and money* and lowers morale.

Unwanted effects should be infrequent with skilled assessment, and well-trained or closely supervised therapists.

Training of Psychotherapists

Therapists usually train following initial qualification and experience in another profession such as psychiatry, psychology, nursing, other health care disciplines and social work. Training requirements vary widely according to the school of therapy, and a period of personal therapy is required by some. Desirable qualities in a therapist are the ability to be sympathetic but detached, non-judgemental, and honest. Therapy is more likely to be successful if patient and therapist like one another, so that a strong "therapeutic alliance" can develop.

NHS Provision of Psychotherapy

Most mental health care services are organised around particular clinical problems and/or patient groups; only Departments of Psychotherapy are based around a particular form of treatment. This somewhat "special" status has extended to the type of psychotherapy offered, which until recently was mainly psychodynamic, carrying considerable prestige and exerting a strong influence on psychiatric education and training.

Recent years have seen a reaction against psychodynamic psychotherapy. Prospective randomised controlled trials have not generally shown superiority of this treatment over comparison conditions, such as waiting list controls. Brief structured psychotherapies of the cognitive and cognitive-behavioural types do, in contrast, appear more effective than control conditions. The recent trends are therefore towards increased use of, and funding for, the latter types. It seems reasonable that health care resources should be focused on treatments which have been shown to be effective ("evidence-based medicine"), especially considering the greater cost of long courses of dynamic therapy. However, part of this movement may represent another swing of the biological/psychological pendulum in the history of psychiatry; too marked a shift away from the fascinating, if "unscientific", notions of psychodynamic psychotherapy may in the future be seen as counterproductive.

Planning and Practical Organisation of Therapy

NHS psychotherapy sessions usually take place weekly and last 50 minutes. All sessions should preferably be at the same time on the same day of the week and in the same place. Punctuality by both patient and therapist is important. Interruptions, including phone calls, should be prevented. These practical rules provide patients with a secure framework in which to explore difficult issues.

Some therapists draw up a contract at the beginning to specify the patient's problems, goals of treatment, and proposed number of sessions.

Notes are written immediately afterwards, but not during the session itself. Details of the content of sessions should not be revealed to other people except in the context of supervision seminars.

Some individual types of psychotherapy will now be described.

COGNITIVE AND COGNITIVE-BEHAVIOURAL THERAPY

Cognitive (Latin *cogito:* I think) therapy is based on the principle that thought influences mood, so that depression, anxiety and other symptoms arise from, or are perpetuated by, faulty thought patterns and beliefs. The aim in therapy is to identify *automatic negative thoughts* which appear to be contributing to the symptoms, and encouraging the patient to reconsider them in the light of the evidence, and to try alternative viewpoints and behaviour patterns. This process should lead to better understanding of the symptoms, and more control over them. For some patients, exploration of visual images is an appropriate variant of this technique.

Beck originally described several types of maladaptive thinking patterns to be addressed in therapy, including:

- *Selective abstraction*: dwelling on only the negative aspects of a situation.
- *Overgeneralisation*: a single matter is wrongly assumed to have wide-ranging implications.
- *Magnification*: a trivial matter is exaggerated out of proportion.
- *All-or-none reasoning*: issues are seen as "black or white" with no middle ground.
- *Arbitrary inference*: things are assumed, without good evidence, to be negative.

Most cognitive therapists are happy to admit that their treatment involves components of behaviour therapy (see below), for example activity scheduling, and that the term cognitive therapy is effectively shorthand for cognitive-behavioural therapy.

Cognitive therapy is brief (6–12 sessions), problem-oriented, and demands active participation both from the therapist, who provides a structured approach and sometimes a substantial educational input, and from the patient.

Structure is provided by several factors, including:

- Prior agreement on the *number of sessions*.
- Setting of *agreed, tangible goals* (such as a patient with social phobia going shopping alone).
- *Planned structure* for each session.
- *Homework*.

A typical session includes:

- Greeting.
- Setting agenda for session.
- Review of homework.
- Review of events since previous session.
- Feedback on last session.
- Problems to be addressed in session.
- Setting homework.
- Feedback.

Components of the therapy include:

- *Cognitive techniques*, for example:
  - questioning negative automatic thoughts
  - distraction techniques to take the patient's attention away from negative thoughts.
- *Behavioural techniques*:
  - keeping a diary: simple notes on thoughts/feelings/activity to establish the influence of thoughts on mood
  - activity scheduling: planning pleasurable experiences/activities.

Many of these are first tried out within the session, and then practised as agreed specific homework tasks.

The skill of the cognitive therapist lies not only in using these techniques and structures, but doing so in a sensitive and supportive way, for the building of a good rapport between patient and therapist is as essential here as in all kinds of therapy. Trust in the therapist will encourage the patient to engage in prescribed tasks which are often anxiety-provoking or even unpleasant in themselves, such as going out for the socially phobic person, or challenging a negative self-concept for the depressed.

Indications

Randomised controlled trials have shown that cognitive-behavioural therapy is as effective as antidepressant drugs in the acute treatment of outpatient, unipolar depressives. Other trials have shown it to be effective for anxiety disorders, bulimia nervosa, somatoform disorders, personality disorders, and maladaptive reactions to physical illness. As well as treating an index episode, this therapy may have prophylactic value in preventing future episodes (secondary prevention).

Case Example

A man who had been made redundant from his job as a bank manager developed a depressive illness; retaining his occupational health insurance for a limited time, he saw a psychiatrist privately. Declining medication, he was referred for cognitive therapy; the insurer agreed to pay for 10 one-hour sessions. The patient considered himself an utter failure at work, and extended this belief to all other aspects of his life (overgeneralisation), perceiving rejections where none were intended and becoming even more depressed in consequence. Objective consideration revealed that his redundancy was one of many in the bank, occasioned by financial difficulties and mechanisation, rather than a personal rejection as he had assumed (arbitrary inference). Keeping a mood diary quickly convinced him of the connection between his thoughts and his depressed mood. He made rapid progress in the first three sessions, but then "got stuck". Further cognitive work increased his insight but did not improve his mood. The therapist noticed his reluctance to set practical goals, and placed more emphasis on activity scheduling, especially pleasurable activities outside the home. By the end of therapy he had made further progress, and was happy with the outcome: patient and therapist agreed that residual symptoms (mainly social anxiety, lack of energy, and poor concentration) would continue to improve if he continued to practise the new thinking skills he had learnt, and to build up his social activities, which had previously been mainly related to his work.

BEHAVIOUR THERAPY

Behaviour therapy is based on learning theory, a model of human and animal behaviour originating in the field of pure (non-clinical) psychology. In the 1950s, workers such as Eysenck, Lazarus, Wolpe, Bandura, Marks and Rachman began to introduce these ideas into clinical practice as behaviour therapy. This involves the acquisition of desirable new behaviours as well as the loss of unwanted ones.

Behaviour therapy was originally applied to those neurotic symptoms which could be regarded as "maladaptive learned responses", for example a monophobia (a phobia restricted to one specific object or situation) developing after a frightening experience. Behavioural techniques have since been applied to a much wider range of disorders, for example generalised anxiety states, obsessive-compulsive disorders, eating disorders, sexual problems, and the management of chronic disability caused by brain damage or schizophrenia.

Problems are defined, and objectives of therapy agreed, at the beginning. Progress during therapy is regularly assessed using measurable criteria: frequency of occurrence of a particular behaviour pattern, questionnaires to monitor mood change, or psychophysiological variables.

Critics have claimed on theoretical grounds that, because the past events or unconscious conflicts which produced the symptoms are ignored, behaviour therapy cannot produce a lasting cure and that "symptom substitution" will occur. In practice this seldom happens.

Behaviour therapy appears comparable in efficacy to other forms of psychotherapy, is often less time-consuming than other methods, and the patient need not be intelligent or verbally fluent to benefit.

Specific techniques include:

- *Systematic desensitisation (graded exposure)*: progressive introduction to a feared object or situation, using an agreed hierarchy. For example, a person with a fear of spiders agrees with the therapist to encounter them first in imagination, then pictures, followed by a plastic one and then a real one.
- *Flooding*: immediate exposure to the feared stimulus in its full form. This is claimed to be as effective as graded exposure, but many patients find the prospect unacceptable.
- *Modelling*: the patient imitates the therapist's behaviour, for example in social skills or assertiveness training.

- *Biofeedback techniques*: to modify physiological variables such as heart rate, blood pressure and muscle tension. Some people find this helpful in controlling anxiety or pain.
- *Response prevention*: for compulsive behaviour. For example, the therapist prevents the obsessional patient from repeated hand-washing; the patient's anxiety initially rises, but then decays naturally when the feared consequence (such as infection) does not occur.
- *Thought stopping*: for obsessional thoughts. The patient learns to stop an obsessional train of thought, usually by "switching" to another. This is very similar to the cognitive technique of "distraction".
- *Massed practice (satiation)*: the unwanted behaviour is repeated so often that the patient no longer wants to continue it.
- *Aversion therapy*: traditional forms are now seldom used for ethical reasons. They involved coupling an unwanted behaviour, such as substance misuse or deviant sexuality, with an unpleasant stimulus such as drug-induced vomiting or electric shock. Milder self-administered forms may be helpful, for example snapping an elastic band worn around the wrist can provide distraction from obsessional thoughts or from an unwanted behaviour such as overeating.
- *Covert sensitisation*: aversion therapy carried out in imagination only.
- *Shaping (chaining)*: the separate learning of each stage in a complex process, for example a brain-damaged or learning-disabled patient learning to dress.
- *Token economy regimes*: rewards are given for desirable behaviour, and privileges withdrawn for undesirable behaviour. The approach has been used in the rehabilitation of chronic schizophrenics, but ethical considerations apply.
- *Relaxation training*: used in a variety of problems, mainly to manage anxiety. The patient tenses up and then progressively relaxes all muscle groups, while breathing regularly and deeply. This is a gradually acquired skill, which can be taught individually or in groups, or with the aid of commercially available audio- and video-tapes.

A course of behaviour therapy would typically involve several of the above components, for example a spider phobic might take part in a programme of graded exposure, and be given relaxation training to cope with attendant anxiety.

It seems likely that most behavioural treatments include some cognitive component, though some purists might not accept this.

PSYCHODYNAMIC PSYCHOTHERAPY

Assessment

Before a patient is taken on for psychodynamic therapy, a detailed initial assessment should be carried out by an experienced therapist. Presenting symptoms should be considered in the light of early experience, use of psychological defence mechanisms, and personality traits. Subsequent treatment may, in training units, be carried out by a more junior therapist under supervision. Duration of treatment in the NHS, previously a year or more, now tends to be measured in months.

Technique, and Mechanisms of Change

The therapist should take the role of a professional but sympathetic listener; avoid asking too many questions; and avoid imposing his or her own feelings and opinions through making moral judgements or giving direct advice. In contrast to cognitive and behavioural therapies, there is no explicit planned agenda to the sessions.

While improvement of current symptoms may result simply from the opportunity to talk and express feelings, more fundamental change usually requires the use of interpretations designed to help the patient be more aware of emotions and express them more clearly:

- *Identifying and challenging defences* against unacknowledged feelings: use of mental defence mechanisms (see Glossary).
- *Pointing out discrepancies* between stated wishes and actual behaviour, for example a patient may repeatedly say that he wishes to end an unsatisfactory relationship, but takes no practical steps to do so.
- *Pointing out links* between earlier life experiences and current problems, for example, a patient's silence in the face of marital problems might parallel his response as a child to difficulties between his parents.
- *Comments on the transference* between patient and therapist as revealed by the patient's behaviour within the session itself. Transference means the patient feels and behaves towards the therapist as towards important figures in the past. Transference can develop more easily if the therapist's real personal attitudes and circumstances are not revealed.

- *Countertransference*, the therapist's feelings and behaviour towards the patient, may also be utilised constructively if properly recognised. If not recognised, they can hinder the therapy.

Evaluation of Results

As discussed above, randomised controlled trials suggest that psychodynamic therapy has little or no therapeutic effect additional to that of comparison conditions, in contrast to the more structured cognitive and behaviour therapies which have consistently demonstrated positive treatment outcomes. Psychodynamic therapists have responded by pointing out that there are difficulties evaluating the outcome, because:

- Neurotic disorders often remit spontaneously.
- Specific effects of psychotherapeutic technique are difficult to distinguish from non-specific benefits of regular individual attention.
- The content of treatment sessions is difficult to standardise because it varies with the individual characteristics of patient and therapist.
- Benefits of a subtle kind may not be detectable by standard questionnaires.

However, these considerations have not prevented cognitive and behavioural therapy being demonstrated as effective. Perhaps the only valid response is that the outcome criteria are not agreed between the two broad schools of psychotherapy; many psychodynamic patients do not fit into a formal diagnostic category, and may wish for therapy for personal development rather than symptom relief. In either case, it is becoming increasingly hard to justify expenditure of limited NHS psychiatric resources on individual psychodynamic therapy, though it is still available in the private sector.

GROUP THERAPY

Group therapy is more powerful than individual therapy for some patients, and more economical of resources. Groups may use any of the techniques described above, for example analytical, cognitive, behavioural.

Selection of Patients

Selection criteria are similar to those for psychotherapy in general. Group therapy is especially suitable for patients whose main problems concern relationships with others, and patients with a shared problem: alcohol or drug misuse, anxiety, childhood sexual abuse for example. Shy patients who find it difficult to participate in group discussion may not benefit, whereas talkative patients may monopolise a group and arouse hostility from the other members, but a skilled therapist can encourage both types to play a more balanced part.

Role of the Therapist

The therapist should facilitate trust and open disclosure, and encourage regular attendance. Factors likely to impede the group's success, such as dropping-out, lateness, absences, socialisation outside the group, breaches of confidentiality and sub-grouping, should be discouraged.

Some therapists act as detached leaders, others participate more actively. Some groups have two co-therapists, preferably of equal status.

Mechanisms of Change

The same mechanisms operate as in individual therapy, but those treated in groups have the advantage of being able to share their problems and ways of coping with others similarly affected.

Organisation of Therapy

As the introduction of newcomers may retard progress and arouse hostility, "closed" groups with a fixed lifespan and the same members throughout are ideal, if not always practicable. A good size is 5–10 members. Outpatient groups usually meet once a week for 1–2 hours. Groups run on psychoanalytic lines may continue for two years or more. Groups using behavioural or cognitive techniques, for example anxiety management groups, last only 6–12 weeks.

Inpatient units run on "therapeutic community" lines use daily group therapy as the main method of treatment.

FAMILY AND MARITAL THERAPY

Psychiatric symptoms are often exacerbated by a dysfunctional relationship between marriage partners, or within a larger family group. Common problems include:

- *Scapegoating*, in which one family member is automatically blamed for problems.
- Extremes of *authority and dependency.*
- *Ambiguous communication styles.*
- *Family secrets.*
- *Gratification* of one person through the illness of another.
- A *shared stress*, such as bereavement, affecting the whole family.

"Systems theory" has been influential; it views the family as a self-contained system, in which changes in one element are compensated for by complementary changes in others. Thus, problems in one family member can be addressed not only directly, but also by changing the response of the others.

Recent trends within society, for example the replacement of traditional marriage by "serial monogamy", more mothers working outside the home, more men unemployed, and fewer old people in close contact with their children and grandchildren, have influenced the type of presenting problems and expectations of outcome.

Therapy involves regular meetings between family members and therapist(s). As with group therapy, a particular technique can be adopted, but general principles include:

- Encouraging *clear communication* between family members.
- Setting *practical goals* agreed by all parties.
- Emphasising *positive aspects* of relationships, and encouraging rewarding behaviour.
- Discouraging *criticisms*, especially repetitive ones about the past.

Role-play may be used to enable better appreciation of others' points of view.

Good motivation by all participants, and a reasonable degree of goodwill and honesty between them, are prerequisites for success and the therapists should avoid taking sides.

FURTHER READING

Books

Barker P (1992) *Basic Family Therapy* (3rd edn). Blackwell Scientific Publications: Oxford

Brown D, Pedder J (1991) *An Introduction to Psychotherapy* (2nd edn). Routledge: London

Hawton K, Salkovskis PM, Kirk J, Clark DM (eds) (1989) *Cognitive Behaviour Therapy for Psychiatric Problems: a Practical Guide.* Oxford University Press: Oxford

Malan DH (1979) *Individual Psychotherapy and the Science of Psychodynamics.* Butterworth-Heinemann: Oxford

Storr A (1990) *The Art of Psychotherapy* (2nd edn). Butterworth Heinemann: Oxford

Review Articles

Andrews (1993) The essential psychotherapies. *British Journal of Psychiatry* **162**: 447–451

Beitman BD, Goldfried MR, Norcross JC (1989) The movement toward integrating the psychotherapies – an overview. *American Journal of Psychiatry* **146**: 138–147

Marks IM (1987) Behavioural psychotherapy in general psychiatry: helping patients to help themselves. *British Journal of Psychiatry* **150**: 593–597

Moorey S (1996) Cognitive behaviour therapy for whom? *Advances in Psychiatric Treatment* **2**: 17–23.

Weissman MM, Markowitz JC (1994) Interpersonal psychotherapy. *Archives of General Psychiatry* **51**: 599–606

23

Psychopharmacology

GENERAL PRINCIPLES ABOUT USING PSYCHOTROPIC DRUGS

Psychotropic drugs are immensely valuable in the treatment of mental illness. They are not, however, a substitute for psychological treatments and social care; best results are often achieved by some combination of all these approaches.

Relevant questions about psychotropic drug use include:

When is drug treatment indicated?
Severe psychiatric illness usually responds well to drugs, but medication may be less effective for milder illness, personality and behaviour disorders and reactions to stress. In primary care, much psychiatric symptomatology is brief and self limiting, and medication not necessary.

Do the therapeutic effects outweigh any negative aspects?
All effective drugs have side-effects, usually but not always unwanted ones. Many psychotropics react adversely with *other drugs*, or with *alcohol*, and impair *driving skills*. *Elderly patients*, women who are *pregnant or breast-feeding*, and *patients with medical disorders* are at greatest risk of unwanted effects. *Tolerance and/or dependence* seldom cause problems except with benzodiazepines, but patients are often

needlessly worried about "getting addicted" to other psychotropics, especially antidepressants. Patients with suicidal tendencies may use psychotropic drugs for *overdose* if issued with large quantities. The *financial cost* of drug treatment is another significant factor, although likely to be considerably less than the cost of inadequately treated mental illness.

If drug treatment seems appropriate but has not worked, has the patient been taking it?

Many patients take their drugs irregularly, or not at all. Compliance can be improved by using single-drug regimes, taken once daily. Most psychotropic drugs persist at therapeutic levels for at least 24 hours, giving little rationale for divided doses.

If drug treatment seems appropriate but has not worked, has the drug been given in adequate dosage for long enough?

Depressive illness treated with antidepressants, and schizophrenia treated with antipsychotics, may take 4–6 weeks to respond. With antidepressants, use of sub-therapeutic doses is a common error.

How long should treatment be continued?

Benzodiazepines for anxiety and insomnia should only be given for a few weeks at a time, because of the risk of tolerance and dependence; but a course of antidepressants, if effective, should be continued several months to prevent relapse. Lithium for prophylaxis of affective disorder, and antipsychotics for maintenance treatment of schizophrenia, are usually continued for several years and sometimes are needed for life.

With difficult or atypical cases it may be necessary to experiment with different pharmacological groups in order to find the best drug, or combination of drugs. Changes should be made one at a time, and not before each one has been given a chance to work.

Which route of administration ?

Oral medication is of course the rule. Liquid rather than solid formulations are easier for some patients to swallow – and harder for uncooperative ones to hide in their mouths. Intramuscular injections include ordinary short-acting ones, for example haloperidol 10 mg for severe agitation in a psychotic patient, and long-acting "depot" preparations where the active medication is esterified and suspended in an oily form from which it is released slowly, for example haloperidol decanoate 100 mg every four weeks to keep chronic schizophrenia in remission. Intravenous injections are rarely used, and are unsafe with some psychotropic drugs.

Proprietary or generic formulation?
Lithium is one of the few psychotropic drugs where this matters pharmacologically, as the same dose of different preparations may produce very different levels in the patient, so the prescriber must specify and stick to a particular one. This consideration does not apply to most other drugs, so generic prescribing to reduce costs is officially encouraged. However, generic prescribing has the disadvantage that different formats (size, shape, colour, taste) of tablets containing the same dose of the same drug are available, causing patients to be alarmed if the appearance of their medication changes when a fresh supply is dispensed.

The need for explanation
Prescription of drugs should always be accompanied by clear explanation and discussion about the need for medication, why a particular compound has been chosen, the likely benefits and risks, and the effects both wanted and unwanted. Such talks take only a short time, are highly valued by patients, and have been shown to improve compliance. Written information leaflets are also helpful.

This chapter describes the main groups of psychotropic drugs, with reference to some commonly used examples: the fuller account in the *British National Formulary* is recommended.

ANTIPSYCHOTICS

Antipsychotics (neuroleptics, major tranquillisers) specifically ameliorate psychotic symptoms (delusions and hallucinations), as well as having a general sedative action. *Chlorpromazine* was first introduced in the 1950s, as an antihistamine; a French surgeon noted its marked sedative action on surgical patients, and it was then tried out on psychiatric patients, often with excellent results. Many other compounds are now available (Box 1).

BOX 1: ANTIPSYCHOTIC DRUGS IN COMMON USE

Generic name	Proprietary name	Chemical group
Chlorpromazine	Largactil	Phenothiazine
Clozapine	Clozaril	Dibenzapine
Droperidol	Droleptan	Butyrophenone
Fluphenazine decanoate*	Modecate	Phenothiazine
Flupenthixol decanoate*	Depixol	Thioxanthene
Fluspirilene*	Redeptin	Diphenylbutylpiperidine
Haloperidol	Serenace	Butyrophenone
Haloperidol decanoate*	Haldol	Butyrophenone
Loxapine	Loxapac	Dibenzapine
Pimozide	Orap	Diphenylbutylpiperidine
Promazine	Sparine	Phenothiazine
Risperidone	Risperdal	Benzisoxazole
Sulpiride	Dolmatil	Benzamide
Thioridazine	Melleril	Phenothiazine
Trifluoperazine	Stelazine	Phenothiazine
Zuclopenthixol decanoate*	Clopixol	Thioxanthene
Zuclopenthixol acetate †	Acuphase	Thioxanthene

* = Long-acting intramuscular injection.
† = Medium-acting intramuscular injection.

Indications

- *Schizophrenia.*
- *Mania.*
- *Severely agitated or violent behaviour* associated with any psychiatric disorder or organic brain syndrome.
- *Anxiety* which has failed to respond to other treatments.
- In general medicine as *antiemetics* and to *potentiate analgesics and anaesthetics.*

Pharmacology

Most antipsychotics are thought to work by blocking D2 receptors in the mesolimbic area of the brain. Serum prolactin level is a measure of this dopaminergic blockade. However, the potent antipsychotic drug *clozapine* does not affect D2 receptors; it may work on D4 or 5-HT receptors instead. Most antipsychotics also block cerebral receptors for noradrenaline. Peripherally they have antiadrenergic, anticholinergic and antihistaminic actions.

Administration

Acute psychosis may be treated with oral medication given three or four times daily, and/or a recently introduced and very useful medium-acting intramuscular preparation, *zuclopenthixol acetate*, which exerts its effects over two to three days. There is a calming effect from the start, but control of delusions and hallucinations may take three or four weeks, and sometimes the full benefit is not seen for six to twelve months. In schizophrenia, the positive symptoms respond better than the negative ones.

Chronic schizophrenia is often treated by slow-release intramuscular injections (depots) every 1–4 weeks. Such injections have a pharmacological advantage for some patients in whom oral medication is incompletely absorbed or undergoes rapid first-pass metabolism in the liver, but their main advantage is ensuring regular medication and follow-up for a group of patients whose compliance with treatment tends to be poor.

For some cases of schizophrenia which do not respond to conventional doses of drugs, high-dose regimens may be effective but their use is controversial because of the risk of potentially fatal cardiac arrhythmias. It may be better to add a drug from another class, usually a benzodiazepine, or consider ECT, before prescribing "megadose" antipsychotics.

Unwanted Effects

Antipsychotic drugs have a great many potential unwanted effects. Most common and troublesome are those involving the *extrapyramidal nervous system*, as follows:

- *Parkinsonism*, with tremor, rigidity, bradykinesia and sialorrhoea
- *akathisia*, with mental agitation and motor restlessness
- *acute dystonia*, including torticollis, other abnormal postures, and oculogyric crisis.

All these extrapyramidal effects respond to *anti-Parkinsonian* drugs such as *benzhexol* or *procyclidine*, but these extra drugs should not be given unless required because they may cause sedation and confusion, exacerbate psychotic symptoms and anticholinergic effects, and also attract drug misusers.

Tardive dyskinesia is another extrapyramidal syndrome which develops in approximately 20% of patients on long-term antipsychotic drug treatment. Elderly, female and brain-damaged patients are most likely to be affected. Involuntary movements of choreiform or athetoid type affect the orofacial muscles, and sometimes the limbs or trunk. The cause may be proliferation or hypersensitivity of dopamine receptors after prolonged blockade by antipsychotic drugs, or imbalance between dopamine and its antagonists acetylcholine and GABA. There is no effective treatment although, paradoxically, increasing the dose of the responsible antipsychotic brings about temporary improvement. Prevention is better, and may be achieved by using the lowest antipsychotic dose which is effective.

Other unwanted effects of antipsychotic drugs include *hypotension, cardiac arrhythmias,* either *dry mouth* or *excessive salivation* (*sialorrhoea*), *constipation, weight gain, reduced fertility, bone marrow depression, blurred vision, retention of urine, impotence, jaundice, rash, photosensitivity,* and *hypothermia* especially in the elderly.

Neuroleptic malignant syndrome is a rare, but potentially fatal, acute complication of antipsychotic drug use. Symptoms include catatonia or extrapyramidal movements, and hyperpyrexia. Affected patients require intensive medical care.

Antipsychotics are mainly metabolised in the liver. Their main drug interaction is to potentiate the sedative effects of other psychoactive substances, most importantly alcohol, antidepressants and benzodiazepines. Liver damage is the main contraindication. Regarding use in pregnancy, no serious adverse effects on the foetus are known. Antipsychotic drugs enter breast milk in small amounts. Antipsychotic drugs lower the convulsive threshold slightly, so caution is required in patients with epilepsy. Tolerance and dependence do not occur.

Choice of Drug

If the first drug chosen does not work, it is logical to change to one of a different chemical group.

Chlorpromazine remains the first-line antipsychotic for many psychiatrists, and the reference with which other drugs are compared. It is more sedating than many others. Chlorpromazine should not be given intravenously because of a risk of cardiac arrhythmias.

Thioridazine causes fewer Parkinsonian effects, but is more likely to cause confusion, because of its strong anticholinergic properties.

Haloperidol is pharmacologically "cleaner" with fewer actions outside the dopaminergic system, but it is very prone to cause extrapyramidal effects.

The newer drugs appear to offer a real advance in the treatment of schizophrenia. *Risperidone* has strong antipsychotic properties but few extrapyramidal effects. *Clozapine* is also a highly effective antipsychotic but is licensed only for use in resistant cases which have failed to respond to first-line drugs, and because of the risk of agranulocytosis is only available on a named-patient basis on condition that regular blood counts are satisfactory. The full benefit of clozapine may not be seen for at least a year.

ANTIDEPRESSANTS: TRICYCLIC GROUP

Tricyclics are the standard first-line drug treatment for depressive illness. *Imipramine* and *amitriptyline* are the longest established drugs of the tricyclic group but many others exist (Box 2), some having a tetracyclic or other chemical structure.

Indications

- *Depressive illness.*
- *Depression* associated with other psychiatric conditions.
- *Anxiety states* and *panic disorder.*
- *Nocturnal enuresis.*
- *Chronic pain,* especially of "neuropathic" type.

BOX 2: TRICYCLIC AND RELATED ANTIDEPRESSANTS IN COMMON USE

Generic name	Proprietary name	Structure
Amitriptyline	Tryptizol	Tricyclic
Clomipramine	Anafranil	Tricyclic
Dothiepin	Prothiaden	Tricyclic
Doxepin	Sinequan	Tricyclic
Imipramine	Tofranil	Tricyclic
Lofepramine	Gamanil	Tricyclic
Maprotiline	Ludiomil	Tetracyclic
Mianserin	Bolvidon, Norval	Tetracyclic
Nortriptyline	Allegron	Tricyclic
Trazadone	Molipaxin	Novel
Trimipramine	Surmontil	Tricyclic

Pharmacology

One mechanism of antidepressant action is believed to be prevention of reuptake of amine neurotransmitters into neurones. Changes in the number or sensitivity of postsynaptic receptors may also be involved. Most antidepressants affect both noradrenaline and 5-HT systems but others act selectively on one or the other. They have peripheral anticholinergic effects.

Administration

These drugs should be started in a small dose, increased every few days if well tolerated. The oral route is almost always used; some parenteral preparations exist but do not have any clear advantage. It is often possible to give the total dose at night; this helps with sleep, and improves compliance. There may be a delay of two or more weeks before the antidepressant effect is manifest and it is essential to counsel patients about this, especially as side-effects are most prominent in the first week. Many patients in fact begin to improve within days rather than weeks, which may be due to the anxiolytic and hypnotic effects of these drugs.

Even if a depressive episode seems to have recovered completely with drug treatment, the drug should be continued in full therapeutic dose for at least six months before being gradually tapered off.

Unwanted Effects

A long list of possible unwanted effects, many of them due to tricyclics' anticholinergic properties, are listed but in practice only a few commonly occur.

Sedation may be beneficial if the patient is anxious or sleeping badly, but can be a nuisance during the day. Affected patients must be advised not to drive or use machinery. Sedation is made worse by alcohol.

Dry mouth, *blurred vision* and *constipation* are common, and *urinary retention* may occur. *Postural hypotension* may be dose-limiting, especially in the elderly. Tricyclics can also cause *confusion* in elderly patients, or those with organic brain disease. Tricyclics lower the *convulsive threshold*, but this effect should not stop their use in a depressed epileptic, where the benefits of effective treatment far outweigh the risk of precipitating a fit.

Less commonly, tricyclics, especially amitriptyline, can cause *cardiac arrhythmias* or *heart block*, precipitating sudden death in some patients with cardiac disease. Other rare but potentially serious effects are precipitation of *glaucoma*, and *hepatic* and *haematological* reactions.

Weight gain is common, and deters some patients from taking these drugs.

Tricyclics are metabolised in the liver. They have additive interactions with monoamine oxidase inhibitors, barbiturates, phenothiazines, anticholinergics, and anticoagulants, also with alcohol. The main contraindications are cardiac disease, glaucoma, and prostatic enlargement. Use in pregnancy is relatively safe as no serious adverse effects on the foetus are known, and tricyclics enter breast milk in small amounts only. Tolerance and dependence are not a significant problem, and it is important to reassure patients of this; however, sudden withdrawal of a tricyclic may cause nausea, headache, sweating and insomnia.

Choice of Drug

Patients in whom depression is accompanied by agitation or insomnia are most likely to benefit from one of the more sedative tricyclics such as *amitriptyline, dothiepin* or *trimipramine,* whereas patients with psychomotor retardation may be better on a non-sedating drug such as *imipramine, lofepramine* or *nortriptyline.*

The side-effect profile may determine the choice of drug, especially in patients with co-existing medical disorders. Compounds such as *amitriptyline* tend to produce more unwanted effects than the newer ones, yet for some patients appear to be more effective as antidepressants.

If depression proves resistant to tricyclics, another drug may be added. *Lithium* augmentation is sometimes helpful. Combined therapy using a tricyclic together with an *SSRI* or *MAOI* (see below) is another option but may be hazardous, so should only be used by experienced specialists.

ANTIDEPRESSANTS: SSRI GROUP

SSRIs (selective serotonin reuptake inhibitors) (Box 3) have been available on the UK market since 1989.

BOX 3: SSRI ANTIDEPRESSANTS

Generic name	*Proprietary name*
Fluoxetine	Prozac
Fluvoxamine	Faverin
Paroxetine	Seroxat
Sertraline	Lustral
Citalopram	Cipramil

SSRIs have been vigorously promoted, and their use is increasing. There is currently much debate about whether they should replace the tricyclics as standard first-line treatment for depressive illness, on the basis of claimed therapeutic advantages which have not always stood up to critical examination. Points of comparison include:

Efficacy: clinical trials suggest that SSRIs and tricyclics are about equal in their antidepressant properties, although some patients will respond better to one or other type of drug. Some psychiatrists have observed that severely depressed patients, especially those whose sleep is disturbed, respond better to a sedative tricyclic such as amitriptyline than to an SSRI.

Unwanted effects: SSRIs are claimed to have fewer unwanted effects than tricyclics but one recent systematic review showed no overall difference. Specifically, SSRIs do not cause anticholinergic effects, cardiotoxicity or weight gain. However they may cause nausea, diarrhoea, anxiety, and loss of weight. Impairment of driving skills is less than with tricyclics. There have been reports that fluoxetine can precipitate violent or suicidal behaviour; whether this is a real risk is not clear. Because SSRIs are still new drugs, any long-term toxicity is not yet known. There is some concern about dependence with paroxetine.

Metabolism: fluoxetine has a very long half-life; this is a disadvantage as far as drug interactions are concerned, but means the drug can be given in one dose every few days as a "depot antidepressant" when compliance is limited.

Safety in overdose: SSRIs are safe in overdosage. Most tricyclics, with the exception of lofepramine, are toxic, and so SSRIs are increasingly used in suicidal patients. However, although tricyclic poisoning is a contributory factor in some suicides, it has never been shown that the total death rate is greater in patients on these more poisonous drugs.

Cost: SSRIs are considerably more expensive.

Dosage: SSRIs have a narrower therapeutic range, and therefore the advantage of a simple standard dose regime, especially useful in the elderly. However, the wide possible dose range of the tricyclics can also be useful, for example in permitting a very small starting dose in a patient susceptible to side-effects.

Other indications: certain SSRIs are licensed for use in eating disorders, panic disorder and obsessive-compulsive disorders, as well as for depressive illness. Fluoxetine has been widely used in the USA to enhance mood, and boost confidence, in people without formal psychiatric disorder; this practice is controversial.

Related antidepressants new to the market are *Venlafaxine* (a *serotonin noradrenaline reuptake inhibitor* or *SNRI*) and *Nefazodone*.

ANTIDEPRESSANTS: MAOI GROUP

MAOIs (*monoamine oxidase inhibitors*) increase brain concentrations of monoamine neurotransmitters by inhibiting the enzymes concerned in their breakdown. They are effective for depression, anxiety and phobic states, and sometimes achieve dramatic responses in patients who have failed to respond to tricyclics.

BOX 4: MAOI ANTIDEPRESSANTS

Generic name	Proprietary name
Isocarboxazid	Marplan
Moclobemide	Mannerix
Phenelzine	Nardil
Tranylcypromine	Parnate

In addition to their anticholinergic side-effects (similar to those described above for the tricyclics), MAOIs may cause potentially dangerous interactions with sympathomimetic drugs and tyramine-containing foods (Box 5). Such interactions produce headache and palpitations and, rarely, a hypertensive crisis leading to a stroke or sudden death. Patients on MAOIs should be given a card listing the items to avoid. It is probable that the risks have been overestimated, and that these effective drugs have been underused as a result. The most recently introduced MAOI, moclobemide, is less prone to cause food and drug interactions because it is selective for the MAO-A isoform, which is found in the liver as opposed to the gut.

BOX 5: INTERACTIONS WITH MAOIs

Drugs	Foods
SSRIs	Cheese (strong)
Amphetamines	Red wine (espec. Chianti)
L-Dopa	Beer (strong)
Fenfluramine	Game
Local anaesthetics	Smoked fish
Ephedrine	"Marmite", "Bovril"

BENZODIAZEPINES

Benzodiazepines were widely prescribed in the 1960s and 1970s as anxiolytics and hypnotics. For a while they were perceived as "wonder drugs" against neurosis, with no side-effects or addiction potential, in contrast to their predecessors the barbiturates. In the 1980s, however, because of concern about their inappropriate use for people with social and interpersonal problems rather than true psychiatric disorder, and because of the risk of dependence, prescription of benzodiazepines was discouraged, with psychological techniques of anxiety management being recommended as an alternative.

BOX 6: BENZODIAZEPINES IN COMMON USE

Generic name	Proprietary name
Alprazolam	Xanax
Chlordiazepoxide	Librium
Diazepam	Valium
Flurazepam	Dalmane
Nitazepam	Mogadon
Lorazepam	Ativan
Temazepam	Normison

At present, benzodiazepines as effective remedies for short-term anxiety are probably underused. Excessive prescription should certainly be avoided, but some authorities consider these drugs a reasonable long-term treatment for a minority of chronically anxious patients. Intensive effort to wean all long-term users off benzodiazepines is not automatically justified.

Further concern about benzodiazepines stems from their popularity with drug misusers. Intravenous injection of the gel from temazepam capsules has recently become prevalent and may cause gangrene of the limbs; these capsules have therefore just been withdrawn.

Indications

- Short-term treatment of *pathological anxiety*.
- Short-term treatment of *insomnia*.
- *Alcohol withdrawal states*.
- *Status epilepticus*.
- *Muscle spasticity*.
- *Anaesthetic premedication*.
- Sedation in *terminal illness*.

Pharmacology

Benzodiazepines probably act through modification of the GABA and glycine neurotransmitter systems in the limbic system and spinal cord.

Administration

Benzodiazepines for anxiety or insomnia are most effective if taken only when required, rather than on a fixed dose regime, and only for a few weeks at a time.

Intramuscular, intravenous and rectal preparations are available for emergency use.

Unwanted Effects

Benzodiazepines, even in overdose, have few unwanted effects in the young healthy person, but the elderly may experience marked side-effects of which neurological and psychiatric ones are most important. These include *confusion, depression, drowsiness, amnesia, impaired psychomotor performance including an effect on driving, ataxia, dysarthria and headache.* Some subjects experience "paradoxical" effects of *excitement, aggression or insomnia. Hallucinations* of a sexual nature have been reported after intravenous benzodiazepine use and may give rise to false accusations of sexual abuse. Benzodiazepines potentiate the effects of alcohol and other cerebral depressants.

Use in *pregnancy* should be avoided. In late pregnancy, benzodiazepines can cause the "floppy infant syndrome" of hypotonia, respiratory embarrassment and hypothermia, and the baby may develop withdrawal symptoms after delivery. Benzodiazepines readily enter breast milk.

Tolerance and dependence may develop with regular use. *Psychological dependence* is common. *Physical dependence* develops in around 20% of those who take benzodiazepines long-term. Suddenly stopping the drugs in such patients causes a withdrawal syndrome of insomnia, tremor, fits, anorexia, vomiting, sweating and cramps. This syndrome, which is most often seen after the withdrawal of a short-acting drug such as *alprazolam, lorazepam* or *temazepam,* may be mistaken for recurrence of the original anxiety for which the drug was prescribed. Withdrawal symptoms can be avoided by tapering the drug gradually, while introducing psychological anxiety management techniques. Some authorities recommend converting the benzodiazepine-dependent patient to the equivalent dose of *diazepam,* which can then be reduced by 1 mg per week over a period of 1–12 months.

Choice of Drug

Many benzodiazepines are available. They vary in potency and duration of action but many are metabolised to the same compound, *oxazepam,* and are to some extent interchangeable. The same compound can often be used in low dose to treat anxiety and in higher dose to induce sleep.

Longer-acting ones can be given in a single night-time dose to provide an immediate hypnotic effect followed by an anxiolytic effect next day. The shorter-acting ones are suitable for insomnia which is not accompanied by day-time anxiety, or for phobic anxiety related to specific situations.

Other Drugs for Anxiety and Insomnia

Various alternatives to the benzodiazepines are available as hypnotics and/or anxiolytics, though all have unwanted effects of their own. *Antidepressants* are often used to treat chronic anxiety, or anxiety mixed with depression. *Amitriptyline, dothiepin* or the newer, less toxic *trazodone* are suitable. Some immediate benefit may occur due to the sedative action, and gradual further improvement should follow over several weeks. Other options include *beta-blockers* such as *propranolol*, effective mainly for the physical symptoms of anxiety; *antipsychotics* such as *thioridazine* in low dose; and newer preparations such as *buspirone*.

For insomnia, long-established remedies include *chloral hydrate* and *promethazine*; newer drugs include *zolpidem* and *zopiclone*. Hypnotics are recommended for occasional use only; dealing with the cause of the insomnia is a better alternative to drugs. Causes include noise, discomfort, a restless partner, worry, shift-work, travel, excess alcohol or caffeine intake, or unrealistic expectations about the amount of sleep required.

Barbiturates, once widely used as hypnotics and anxiolytics before benzodiazepines became available, are now obsolete as psychotropic drugs because of the high risk of dependence and high toxicity in overdose.

LITHIUM

Lithium is the lightest of the alkali metals.

Indications

- *Prophylaxis of recurrent episodes of affective disorder*, when these are sufficiently frequent or disabling to justify long-term continuous drug treatment. In the past, lithium has been used mainly in bipolar disorder, being effective in reducing both frequency and severity of episodes. Lithium is now increasingly used in prophylaxis of recurrent unipolar depression also.
- *Adjunctive treatment of episodes of mania and depression.*
- *Schizophrenia*, especially of *schizoaffective* type.
- *Aggressive* and *self-mutilating* behaviour.

Administration

Although any one of lithium's soluble salts could potentially be used, only the carbonate and citrate are marketed. Plain lithium carbonate must be given three times daily to produce a steady serum level, but slow-release tablets for once-daily administration are available. No parenteral preparations exist.

Therapeutic effect is related to serum lithium level. Levels of 0.8–1.2 mmol/litre are traditionally recommended for prophylaxis, but some patients are controlled on lower levels of 0.5–0.8 mmol/litre. Higher levels may be required for treatment of mania, but toxic effects are likely above 1.5 mmol/litre.

Lithium has a narrow therapeutic margin, and there is individual variation in the dosage needed to produce a given serum level, so regular measurements are required. Blood for serum lithium should be taken eight hours after the last dose. Blood tests are recommended weekly for the first four weeks of therapy, then monthly for a year, then three-monthly. Extra tests should be performed in the event of a change in the preparation or in dosage; if symptoms suggesting lithium toxicity develop; intercurrent illness; or prescription of additional drugs which may interact, especially diuretics.

Thyroid, renal and cardiac function should be assessed before starting lithium and then annually.

If a patient has remained free of depression or mania for some years, it is reasonable to try gradual withdrawal of lithium, as the illness may have undergone a natural remission.

Unwanted Effects

- Relatively harmless: *nausea, mild diarrhoea, fine tremor* (which can be treated by a beta-blocker), *weight gain, oedema,* and *exacerbation of psoriasis.*
- Acute symptoms suggesting *lithium intoxication: vomiting, diarrhoea, coarse tremor, drowsiness, vertigo, dysarthria* and *cardiac arrhythmias.* This condition is serious and, if such symptoms develop, lithium should be stopped immediately and blood taken for estimation of the serum level.
- Long-term effects of gradual onset: *hypothyroidism* (affecting 3% of patients per year, usually reversible when the drug is stopped, and treatable with thyroxine if lithium is continued); rarely, *thyrotoxicosis;* histological and functional changes in the *kidney,* of uncertain significance; and possibly *memory impairment,* and *suppression of creativity.*

Case Example

A postgraduate student, 23 years old, presented with an episode of psychotic depression which responded well to inpatient treatment, but he developed a manic illness some months later. He was started on lithium, but stopped taking it after a few days, complaining of tremor; he had also, through a doctor relative, found out about its unwanted effects, and felt that these had not been properly discussed with him. He recovered, but had a further severe manic episode one year later. This time, he responded only slowly to antipsychotic medication, and lithium was added with gradual success.

Despite repeated discussions, he continued to refuse long-term lithium prophylaxis on the grounds of his fears about unwanted effects, until he was put in touch with a fellow patient with bipolar disorder who had benefited greatly from this treatment for several years, finding it generally harmless when properly supervised. He then took lithium for several years; he continued to have affective episodes approximately annually, though they were less severe and able to be managed without inpatient admission. He came to accept his slight fine tremor as the price of his mental stability.

Lithium should only be used in low dose, and under frequent supervision, in patients with *cardiac or renal impairment, thyroid disease, diabetes insipidus, Addison's disease, obesity,* or on *diuretic therapy.* Neurological impairment after combined dosage with lithium and haloperidol in high dose has been reported. Use in *early pregnancy* is teratogenic, the most common foetal malformation affecting the tricuspid valve of the heart. This and other deformities can be detected by ultrasound. After the first trimester, lithium is believed to be safe, and may need to be continued in women with severe manic-depressive illness although the drug should be stopped for a few days at the time of delivery because of the risk of toxicity. Lithium enters breast milk.

Carbamazepine, widely used as an anticonvulsant and for other indications such as atypical facial pain, is an alternative for prophylaxis of affective disorder, being more effective or better tolerated than lithium in some patients. As with lithium, regular measurements of serum levels are necessary to make sure they are within the therapeutic range. In resistant cases, lithium and carbamazepine can be used together.

FURTHER READING

Books

British National Formulary. Published in frequently updated editions by British Medical Association and Royal Pharmaceutical Society of Great Britain.

Cookson J, Crammer J, Heine B (1993) *The Use of Drugs in Psychiatry* (4th edn). Gaskell: London

King D (ed) (1995) *Seminars in Psychopharmacology.* Gaskell Books: London

Review Articles

Ballinger BR (1990) Hypnotics and anxiolytics. *British Medical Journal* **300**: 456–458

Edwards JG (1992) Selective serotonin reuptake inhibitors. *British Medical Journal* **304**: 1644–1646

Ferrrier IN, Tyrer SP, Bell AJ (1995) Lithium therapy. *Advances in Psychiatric Treatment* **1**: 102–108

Kerwin RW (1994) The new atypical antipsychotics. *British Journal of Psychiatry* **164**: 141–148

Price LH, Heninger GR (1994) Lithium in the treatment of mood disorders. *New England Journal of Medicine* **331**: 591–598

Thompson C (1994) The use of high-dose antipsychotic medication. *British Journal of Psychiatry* **164**: 448–458

Tyrer P, Murphy S (1987) The place of benzodiazepines in psychiatric practice. *British Journal of Psychiatry* **151**: 719–723

24

Electroconvulsive Therapy

Electroconvulsive Therapy (ECT) introduced by Cerletti in Italy in 1938, involves production of a fit by passing an electric current through the brain. ECT today is carried out under a short general anaesthetic, and a muscle relaxant is given to reduce the intensity of the fit. Modern ECT machines deliver brief square-wave (not sine-wave) pulses of electricity and allow the "dose" to be individually adjusted for the patient.

Though ECT has always tended to arouse controversy, with some pressure groups demanding a ban on its use, most psychiatrists consider it a highly effective and sometimes lifesaving treatment for certain severe mental illnesses.

INDICATIONS

Depressive illness is the main indication. An MRC research study in 1965 showed that ECT is superior to antidepressant drugs for treating severe depression. Most depressed patients, however, are given drugs as the first-line treatment with ECT being used in the following circumstances:

- When life is threatened by *suicidality*.
- When life and health are threatened by *refusal of food and drink*.
- When antidepressant *drugs have failed*.
- When antidepressant *drugs are contraindicated* for medical reasons, such as cardiac arrhythmias.

- In the *elderly*, including some with cognitive impairment, when unwanted effects of medication may make drug treatment slower and riskier.
- Occasionally in *palliative care*, when a quick response is needed in someone with not long to live and already on multiple medications.

ECT is occasionally used for inpatients with severe *schizophrenia*, especially *catatonic schizophrenia*, or *mania* which has not responded to intensive drug treatment. ECT is probably underused in such cases, for it often has good results, and may well be safer than large doses of psychotropic medication.

MODE OF ACTION

This is unknown, but may relate to alterations in neurotransmitter sensitivity. ECT causes many physiological changes, including slowing of the EEG, and increased secretion of sympathetic amines, prolactin and other pituitary hormones, but none of these correlate reliably with clinical response. Some sceptics claim that ECT is effective because it results in confusion which makes the patient forget depressing thoughts.

Production of an adequate fit, arbitrarily defined as a generalised tonic-clonic seizure lasting at least 25 seconds, appears to be necessary for a good clinical effect. The minimum size of electrical stimulus required to cause a fit varies a great deal between patients, and is influenced by many factors including age, medication, and previous exposure to ECT. Ideally the stimulus should be individually adjusted to be slightly above the individual's seizure threshold. If the stimulus is too low, no fit occurs; if too high, marked confusion may follow the treatment.

Research studies comparing real ECT with "pseudo ECT", in which an anaesthetic and muscle relaxant are given but no electric shock, shows real ECT is more effective in the treatment of depression but "pseudo ECT" has some clinical benefit too. This suggests that factors such as the complexity and mystique of the treatment, the extra medical and nursing attention and/or the anaesthetics, are partly responsible for the therapeutic effect.

EFFICACY AND PREDICTION OF RESPONSE

About 80% of severe depressive episodes respond well to ECT in the short term. Features predicting a good response include retardation, guilt, delusions, early morning waking, symptoms worse in the mornings, short duration of illness and stable premorbid personality.

Milder depression tends not to respond well, especially if mixed with anxiety in a patient with neurotic symptoms and poorly adjusted premorbid personality.

About two-thirds of patients given ECT for depression will relapse within six months, unless given maintenance treatment with an anti-depressant drug or lithium.

TIMING AND NUMBER OF TREATMENTS

ECT is usually given twice a week for depressive illness, and more frequent administration has no advantage. For mania, daily administration may be better.

The number of treatments required in a course of ECT varies considerably, though typically would be 6–10. There is usually a transient improvement for a few hours after each application, which gradually becomes sustained.

Most depressive illnesses are episodes of a recurrent condition, often requiring prophylactic treatment; this is usually with medication, but occasional patients seem to do best with "maintenance" ECT administered every 2–4 weeks.

PRACTICALITIES OF TREATMENT

Treatment is best carried out in a specially equipped ECT suite within a psychiatric unit. Inpatient admission is usual for the first course, but outpatient ECT is feasible for patients in good general health, who can be trusted not to eat or drink on the morning of treatment, and not to drive or cycle home afterwards. The treatment is carried out by a psychiatrist, a nurse and an anaesthetist. Physical examination must be performed before the course begins, in order to exclude the contraindications listed below.

CONTRAINDICATIONS

- *Anaesthetic contraindications* such as severe respiratory or cardiac disease.
- *Organic brain disease* of a kind in which increased cerebral blood flow would be dangerous, such as cerebral aneurysm, or conditions involving raised intracranial pressure. Other forms of organic brain disease including dementia, epilepsy and a past history of head injury do not necessarily rule out the use of ECT, but do carry an increased risk of confusion after treatment.

These contraindications are relative, not absolute, and may need to be balanced against the risk to life posed by severe depression when deciding whether ECT is justified.

Pregnancy is not a contraindication, nor is old age.

BILATERAL vs UNILATERAL ECT

The electrodes may be applied to both sides of the head (bilateral ECT), which is the standard treatment, or to the non-dominant side only (unilateral ECT). Bilateral ECT produces greater memory loss and confusion, but is more effective in that fewer treatments per course are needed for a therapeutic effect. Bilateral ECT is therefore preferred when a rapid response is required, but patients prone to marked cognitive impairment may be better treated with unilateral ECT.

UNWANTED EFFECTS

- *Memory impairment*: transient memory impairment, both retrograde and anterograde, is frequent. A few patients complain of persistent memory loss after ECT, but research studies have found no evidence for long-term cognitive impairment or structural brain changes even after multiple ECT treatments.
- *Confusion*: mild transient confusion after treatment is frequent. If a severe confusional state develops, ECT should be discontinued, and evidence for organic brain disease sought.
- *Anaesthetic complications*.
- *Fractures*: not a hazard if the fit is adequately modified by a muscle relaxant.

- *Mania* may be precipitated when ECT is given to patients with bipolar affective disorder in the depressed phase.

Mortality is 1 per 50 000 treatments, almost always from anaesthetic complications.

CONSENT FOR ECT

Most patients who have ECT do so voluntarily. They are required to sign a consent form before treatment. This should be preceded by a full explanation of the procedure, reinforced by an information leaflet.

Some patients refuse, or are unable to give, informed consent. If such patients appear to be in urgent need of ECT, they may be treated as an emergency either under common law or under Section 62 of the Mental Health Act 1983. However, it is much more usual to apply Section 3 of this Act, and to seek the necessary second opinion from a doctor appointed by the Mental Health Act Commission.

MYTHS

Many patients are horrified when ECT is first suggested. The public perception, reinforced by certain sections of the media, is of "unmodified" ECT as it used to be given thirty years ago without an anaesthetic. There were frequent physical complications such as broken teeth and bones, plus the dehumanising character of the experience, for example patients were often treated one after another in a public ward, with no privacy and no tranquillising medication.

Modern administration of ECT is very different; patients are anaesthetised, treated and recovered in privacy, and complications are rare. Many patients who have been successfully treated with ECT ask for further treatment if their illness recurs. Research has shown that over half those patients who have had ECT consider it less unpleasant than going to the dentist.

FURTHER READING

Books

Abrams R (1992) *Electroconvulsive Therapy* (2nd edn). Oxford University Press: Oxford

Freeman C (1994) *The Practical Administration of ECT* (2nd edn). Royal College of Psychiatrists: London

Review Articles

Lock T (1994) Advances in the practice of electroconvulsive therapy. *Advances in Psychiatric Treatment* **1**: 47–56

Scott AIF (1994) Contemporary practice of electroconvulsive therapy. *British Journal of Hospital Medicine* **51**: 334–339

Video

A video demonstrating the practical administration of ECT is available from the Royal College of Psychiatrists, 17 Belgrave Square, London SW1X 8PG (tel 0171 235 2351)

25

Psychosurgery (Leucotomy, Lobotomy, Functional Neurosurgery)

Psychosurgery is brain surgery carried out to relieve a patient's suffering by changing mood or behaviour.

HISTORY

The history of psychosurgery serves to illustrate the way that the relative influences of the biological and the psychological approaches to psychiatry have varied over time. During the early decades of the twentieth century psychological theories predominated, in particular the various schools of psychoanalysis. However, their results in the treatment of psychiatric patients proved disappointing, particularly in relation to the rapid progress being made in other branches of medicine. This led to a renewed search for what became known as physical treatments (including convulsive therapy, either electrically induced or by chemical means, psychosurgery, insulin coma, electrosleep). Of these methods, only ECT (Ch 24) has been shown effective in prospective randomised controlled trials, and the rest have now fallen out of use. Psychiatrists' enthusiasm for these and other unproven physical treatments, often used without informed consent, was a major reason for the emergence of the "antipsychiatry" movement in the 1960s.

Moniz introduced psychosurgery in Portugal in 1935. During the next twenty years many patients in mental hospitals all over the world underwent lobotomy, entailing large-scale, blind destruction of brain tissue. Some responded well, but others gained no benefit, suffered marked unwanted effects or even died. The introduction in the 1950s of an effective antipsychotic drug (chlorpromazine) was followed by a decline in psychosurgery, although a few specialised centres have continued to carry out operations under strict legal and clinical control, and develop more refined surgical techniques. In England and Wales, only the Brook Hospital in London is now permitted to carry out the procedure; 15–20 operations per year are performed there. In some other countries, psychosurgery has been made illegal.

INDICATIONS

Psychosurgery is reserved as a treatment of last resort for patients with severe longstanding mental illness which has failed to respond to the most vigorous and sustained treatment by other means. The best results are found in the following conditions:

- *Affective disorders*: unipolar or bipolar.
- *Anxiety states*.
- *Obsessive-compulsive disorders*.

Psychosurgery is no longer considered appropriate for some of the other disorders, such as schizophrenia and anorexia nervosa, for which it has been tried in the past.

PREOPERATIVE PREPARATION

- *Thorough trial of conventional treatments*: an intensive, prolonged period of inpatient therapy using a combination of psychotropic drugs, ECT and psychological therapies is mandatory before psychosurgery is considered.
- *Organic brain disease* should be excluded through appropriate investigations including brain scan.

CONSENT

Psychosurgery is one of the few medical treatments where the patient's informed consent is not legally sufficient. Under the Mental Health Act 1983, two independent medical recommendations are also required. This reflects Parliament's concern that this treatment should be closely regulated to prevent the repeat of past abuses.

CONTRAINDICATIONS

- *Personality disorder.*
- *Drug or alcohol misuse.*
- *Organic brain disease.*
- *Severe physical illness* which would increase the operative risk.

OPERATIVE TECHNIQUE

A general anaesthetic is given. A localised brain lesion is created using either radioactive rods (yttrium-90), cutting, freezing, thermo-coagulation or suction. Stereotactic frames ensure accurate localisation. The position chosen for the lesion depends on the psychiatric diagnosis, for example:

- *Subcaudate tractotomy* for affective disorders, anxiety states and obsessive-compulsive disorders.
- *Limbic leucotomy* for obsessive-compulsive disorders.
- *Amygdalotomy* for control of aggression.

AFTERCARE

Severe psychiatric symptoms such as intense suicidal drive or depressive stupor usually recover within days, but other aspects of recovery take longer and it may be up to a year before the full benefits of the operation are apparent. Intensive psychosocial rehabilitation is essential during this time. Psychotropic drugs usually need to be continued.

UNWANTED EFFECTS

Mortality and morbidity are low with modern procedures, but a small risk of serious bleeding or infection does exist. Transient headache and confusion are common in the immediate postoperative period, but recover within a few weeks. Epilepsy develops in about 2% of patients, and can usually be controlled by anticonvulsant drugs. Other side-effects, common with the older operations but rare with modern techniques, include disinhibition, lethargy, intellectual defects, neurological defects, incontinence, weight gain and endocrine changes.

OUTCOME

About 60% of patients are observed to have a good response, but psychosurgery has never been subject to a prospective randomised controlled trial. Its proponents have argued, hitherto successfully, that it would be unethical to randomise in such a trial, though it could equally well be argued that it is unethical to use an unproven treatment.

FURTHER READING

Bridges PK, Bartlett JR, Hale AS, Poynton AM, Malizia AL, Hodgkiss AD (1994) Psychosurgery: stereotactic subcaudate tractotomy. An indispensable treatment. *British Journal of Psychiatry* **165**: 599–611

26

Organisation of Services

BACKGROUND AND HISTORY

Psychiatric disorders require rather different systems of care from physical ones. This is because many psychiatric disorders are chronic; impair patients' ability to meet their own practical and social needs; and often evoke rejection or ridicule from other people, rather than understanding and sympathy.

Until the "asylum movement" of the eighteenth and nineteenth centuries, most mentally ill and mentally handicapped people were looked after by their relatives, with private nursing at home (see *Jane Eyre*, 1847) or in a private "madhouse" for the minority who could afford it. Some were rejected by their families to become "vagrants" and be put in the workhouse, or possibly taken in by religious or charitable institutions. Asylums (hospitals for the mentally ill and mentally handicapped), set up with the help of charitable support amid much initial enthusiasm, were large impressive buildings usually sited in the countryside with their own gardens and farms. However, in the absence of any really effective treatments for psychiatric illness until the mid-twentieth century, their wards soon became overcrowded, and standards and morale declined. Long-stay patients, including many who would not have been considered to merit even a brief psychiatric hospitalisation nowadays, became apathetic and lacking in simple skills of daily living ("institutionalised"). A major stigma was attached to admission.

The gradual closure of asylum beds began in the 1950s, was accelerated in the 1960s and 1970s by several scandals and a fashionable "anti-psychiatry" movement, and has continued to the present day under government policy of "community care".

In the 1970s, many modern inpatient units attached to district general hospitals (DGH units) were built to replace the old mental hospitals. DGH units offered the advantages of enabling psychiatric services to be integrated with medical and surgical ones, close to main centres of population. However the typical DGH unit environment, with its compact unlocked wards, proved unsuitable for certain patients such as the behaviourally disturbed, and accumulation of "new long-stay" cases soon caused blocked beds. The more recent trend has been development of community mental health centres (see below) with the aim of reducing inpatient admissions further still.

In the 1990s, in the context of managerial reorganisation of the NHS as a whole, profound organisational changes to psychiatric services have been introduced, often without pilot studies or prospective evaluation. There is currently much debate as to which model is best, and what future policy should be, and the reader should note that service provision as outlined in this chapter is still evolving, and arrangements vary in different parts of the country.

COMMUNITY CARE

Community care involves treating patients as far as possible in their own homes, with an emphasis on a prompt and individualised multidisciplinary response to problems. Community care is recommended on the grounds that it is as effective as hospital care, preferred by patients and their families, minimises the stigma of mental illness and prevents institutionalisation. These are real advantages provided the systems are well organised, and adequately funded; good community care is not necessarily cheaper than hospital care.

Disadvantages include an increased burden on relatives, and inconvenience or even danger to the general public from behaviour-disturbed or violent patients. There has been much recent concern that, because of underfunding and lack of collaboration between the many professional groups involved, community care programmes are failing, especially in poor inner-city areas. Some patients with severe chronic mental illness have not received proper follow-up, with the result that their clinical state has deteriorated, they live in poor social conditions, and are at increased risk of harming themselves or others. Concern about such cases has led to calls for stricter controls, for example introduction of the Care Programme Approach and Supervision Registers (see below), and provision of more district-based "medium secure" units.

PSYCHIATRY IN PRIMARY CARE

About a quarter of consultations in primary care (general practice) appear to have a substantial psychological component, although the patient's presenting complaint is usually a somatic one and the underlying emotional disturbance may not be recognised by the doctor. Mixed neurotic symptoms, often accompanied by social or interpersonal problems, predominate. About 90% of patients with psychiatric disorder are managed solely in primary care, and many episodes resolve quickly without specific treatment, or with brief counselling; some general practices employ their own counsellors.

Some patients require psychotropic drug therapy. Antidepressants, though often prescribed in lower doses and for shorter courses than most psychiatrists would recommend, are effective. Benzodiazepines are recommended for short periods only.

General practitioners (GPs) are also involved, in collaboration with psychiatric and social services, in the ongoing care of those with more severe illnesses such as schizophrenia and affective disorder which require long-term medication and supervision.

Besides being providers of primary mental health care, GPs are involved in shaping local psychiatric services. Fundholding GPs purchase mental health services for their patients. Fundholding has accelerated the trend towards community psychiatric nurses (CPNs) and other mental health care staff being based in health centres. Concern is sometimes expressed about such specialist resources being directed towards the "worried well", and away from patients with severe chronic psychiatric illness, who may find it difficult even to get registered with a GP in certain areas.

THE PSYCHIATRIC MULTIDISCIPLINARY TEAM

The multidisciplinary team consists of one or more members of each professional group involved in psychiatric patient care: doctors, nurses, clinical psychologists, social workers and occupational therapists. Teams in general adult psychiatry are usually responsible for a defined geographical sector of the health district's catchment area. Other teams, often covering a wider area, deal with specialties such as old age psychiatry, child psychiatry, learning disability, substance misuse, forensic psychiatry, psychotherapy and rehabilitation.

A *community mental health team* may be based in a hospital, a health centre, a converted private house or a purpose-built unit within the community served. Each team member is involved in assessment and management of referred patients, contributing both from their professional viewpoint and from their personal knowledge of the patient. Day-to-day clinical management is often carried out by non-medical team members, but ultimate responsibility for patient care is said to remain with the consultant, or the referring GP.

In some areas, community mental health centres have been set up by social service departments with input from the voluntary sector, especially mental health charities.

INPATIENT SERVICES

Despite the national reduction in psychiatric bed numbers, there still remains a need for some inpatient facilities, whether in a mental hospital, or a DGH unit, or a community unit. Separate wards exist for:

- *Acute admissions in general adult psychiatry* (usually patients aged 18–65). Sometimes there is a separate *intensive care unit* for severely disturbed patients.
- *Acute admissions in old age psychiatry* (patients over 65, or 75). There may be separate wards for functional illness, and for assessment of dementia cases.
- *Medium-stay* and *rehabilitation*.

The above services are required in every health district. They are supplemented by various types of supported accommodation provided by social services (see below).

More specialised inpatient units exist to cover a wider population, such as a health region. These deal with, for example, *forensic cases* (*secure units*), *drug and alcohol misuse, adolescent psychiatry, mother and baby care, eating disorders*.

OUTPATIENT CLINICS

General psychiatric outpatient clinics, mainly conducted by the medical members of the team, exist for assessment and treatment of new referrals, and for follow-up of recent discharges from inpatient care. Many patients do not require indefinite clinic follow-up, but can be discharged to GP care with recommendations for future management.

Some clinic sessions, often supervised by specialist nurses, are dedicated to particular patient groups, for example those on long-term medication with lithium or depot antipsychotics. Computer registers to monitor the frequency of patient attendance, prescribing activity and performance of relevant laboratory tests are a useful aid to managing such clinics and reviewing their performance.

HOME TREATMENT

In a few areas, home treatment has been developed as an alternative to inpatient care for acute cases. This involves a *"crisis intervention"* model in which several members of the multidisciplinary team visit the patient, and family, at frequent intervals sometimes several times per day. While this way of managing acute illness episodes is not yet common practice, there has been a general shift towards providing other interventions in patients' homes, for example domiciliary assessment of new referrals, and regular visits by community psychiatric nurses (CPNs) to monitor patients who need long-term care.

DAY HOSPITALS

Many acutely ill patients can be managed in a Day Hospital as an alternative to admission, and Day Hospitals can also provide a useful period of follow-up care for those recently discharged but still needing intensive support. They offer medical and nursing care, occupational therapy, psychological treatments and social work.

PREVENTING SOCIAL HANDICAP

Severe prolonged psychiatric illness, notably chronic schizophrenia, may lead to loss of daily living skills and/or socially undesirable behaviour. The result may be breakdown of family relationships, homelessness, poverty and unemployment.

Rehabilitation programmes aim to reduce disablement, or better still to prevent this through early intervention; and to improve social functioning and quality of life. This might involve a worthwhile occupation, and a stable social network preferably involving the family, in addition to psychiatric symptom control. A psychiatric rehabilitation team must work closely with social services and community organisations. Individual programmes take account of each patient's impairments, positive attributes, and likely future environment. Progress towards agreed goals is often achieved gradually, over a period of two years or more. The programme may take place in a designated hospital ward or, more often nowadays, in a day care or home setting.

THE CARE PROGRAMME APPROACH

The Care Programme Approach (CPA) was recently introduced by the Department of Health with the aim of improving delivery of services to psychiatric patients. Following a formal assessment of their medical and social needs, patients and carers themselves are invited to take part in drawing up individual written care plans. These might include statements about the frequency of outpatient reviews, medication, home visits by a CPN and/or social work interventions with the family. The resulting document is signed by those responsible. Regular review meetings follow. Although several members of the multidisciplinary team are likely to be involved, the plan must specify a named "key worker" who will coordinate the care, and be the first point of contact in a crisis.

Although the CPA has been introduced and monitored nationally, local providers of care have been left to decide such important aspects as whether it should be applied to all patients or just, for example, those being discharged from inpatient care.

THE SUPERVISION REGISTER

Each district must now keep a Register of psychiatric patients judged to need special supervision on the grounds of risk to themselves or others. This system, recently introduced by the government following adverse publicity over a small number of cases where a mentally disordered person harmed either himself or someone else, has been criticised by many psychiatrists but it is too early to comment on its usefulness.

SOCIAL SERVICES

Community care for patients with long-term mental illness is now the responsibility of local authority social services departments. Each patient (client) must have an individual needs assessment, and then the social worker arranges appropriate services, though clients with sufficient financial means must contribute to the cost of these. As well as general support and advocacy, a social worker will provide advice about:

- *Financial benefit entitlements.*
- *Employment*: for example, sheltered employment, or a gradual return to the work routine through activities in the voluntary sector.
- *Accommodation*: *residential and nursing homes* care for huge numbers of people with mental health problems, not only the elderly. *Group homes, hostels* and other forms of accommodation may be provided by health, social services or the voluntary sector, with varying degrees of resident or non-resident supervision. The *supported lodgings* scheme allows for social services to pay landlords extra in exchange for some care of their tenants. *Private rented accommodation* is home to many with chronic mental illness; some of the landlords involved may be open to criticism, but their tenants might otherwise be homeless.
- *Day centres* provide a focus for regular supervision, activities and rehabilitation.
- *Case management* is a scheme used by some social services departments to improve coordination of care for clients with multiple complex needs. It involves, for example, seeking out someone who fails to attend an appointment. It is much more expensive than standard care, and its clinical effectiveness is unproven.

NON-NHS HEALTHCARE FACILITIES

Although the most psychiatric services are provided by the NHS, some care is purchased from other providers. Examples include:

Private psychiatric hospitals: including some set up for profit, and some non-profit-making charitable institutions. Services from both types are often purchased by the NHS, in areas where it cannot itself meet demand. "Difficult to manage" patients, especially the acutely psychotic and potentially violent; those suffering the chronic effects of brain injury; and special groups such as patients with eating disorders or puerperal illnesses, are among those most frequently placed in the private sector. Many private wards offer higher levels of staffing, and tighter physical security, than most modern NHS facilities.

The voluntary sector: this receives public monies to provide services; for example a charity may receive social services or health funds in order to provide "meals on wheels" or a day centre.

Psychological treatments such as counselling, and various forms of alternative or complementary medicine, are frequently purchased by patients directly. The practitioners consulted may or may not be properly trained and accredited, and patients tend not to reveal this information unless sensitively asked.

FURTHER READING

Books

Pullen I, Wilkinson G, Wright A, Gray DP (eds) (1994) *Psychiatry and General Practice Today*. London: The Royal College of Psychiatrists and the Royal College of General Practitioners

Review Articles

Kingdon D (1994) Making care programming work. *Advances in Psychiatric Treatment* **1**: 41–46

Marks I (1992) Innovations in mental health care delivery. *British Journal of Psychiatry* **160**: 589–597

27

The Mental Health Act 1983

The majority of patients admitted to psychiatric hospitals are voluntary, or informal. The Mental Health Act 1983 (henceforth called "the Act") is concerned with the minority who are unwilling to accept hospitalisation or treatment which others consider essential. Patients in hospital under the Act may be described as "detained" or "sectioned". The general aims of the Act are:

- To provide appropriate care for the mentally disordered.
- To safeguard those who are not mentally disordered against wrongful detention.

Informed use of this legislation should achieve the best possible compromise between preserving freedom and human rights on the one hand, and protecting both patients and society on the other.

The Act gives no authority over those who do not suffer from mental disorder. It cannot be used to enforce treatment for physical illness, unless the physical illness is believed to be causing a mental disorder.

In a life-threatening situation, emergency treatment may be enforced under common law without applying the Act first.

The following summary applies to the legislation for England and Wales. Other countries have separate legislation. The Act is applied in the light of an official Code of Practice, which gives helpful practical guidance on many of the clinical dilemmas which arise.

The Act uses four broad diagnostic categories of mental disorder:

- *Mental illness*, which it does not define.

- *Severe mental impairment*: a state of arrested or incomplete development of mind which includes significant impairment of intelligence and social functioning and is associated with abnormally aggressive or seriously irresponsible conduct on the part of the person concerned.
- *Mental impairment*: as above, except "not amounting to severe mental impairment" is added.
- *Psychopathic disorder*: a persistent disorder or disability of mind (whether or not including significant impairment of intelligence) which results in abnormally aggressive or seriously irresponsible conduct on the part of the person concerned.

Antisocial or immoral conduct, sexual deviancy, and misuse of alcohol or drugs are not sufficient evidence for mental disorder on their own. However, mental disorders caused by substance misuse, for example alcoholic hallucinosis and amphetamine psychosis, are covered by the Act in the usual way.

COMPULSORY ADMISSIONS

For most "Sections", an *application* is made by either an *approved social worker* (ASW) employed by local authority social services, or by the *nearest relative*, on the basis of one or more *medical recommendations*, for the admission of the patient to an approved hospital. In order to prevent collusion within families, the Code of Practice recommends that an ASW rather than a relative is the applicant, and this is almost always the case.

Section 2: Admission for Assessment

Patient: must have a *mental disorder* and detention must be necessary for his/her own health or safety or for the protection of others.
Applicant: ASW/nearest relative.
Medical recommendations: two: one must be approved under Section 12 of the Act and is usually a *psychiatrist*, the other doctor is usually the patient's *general practitioner*.
Duration: up to *28 days*.
Right of appeal: to a Mental Health Tribunal within the first *14 days*, also the nearest relative has the power to discharge the patient from the Section.

Section 3: Admission for Treatment

Patient: must have a *mental disorder* as for Section 2, but if the disorder is *psychopathic disorder* or *mental impairment*, there are further requirements that treatment must be considered likely to *alleviate or prevent deterioration* of the condition. This section permits *treatment*, as well as detention, against the patient's will.
Duration: up to *six months* and then renewable; it must be reviewed before expiry.
Right of appeal: to a Mental Health Review Tribunal within the first *six months*, then once within each renewal period. Review by a tribunal is automatically carried out after six months if the patient has not already applied for a hearing. Renewal is appropriate if treatment is likely to alleviate, or prevent deterioration in, the patient's condition, or (for mental illness or severe mental impairment) the patient, if discharged, would be unlikely to be able to care for himself, or obtain the care he needs, or to guard himself against serious exploitation. The nearest relative can also apply for discharge.

Section 4: Emergency Admission

Patient: as above for Section 2.
Application: nearest relative/ASW.
Recommendation: any one registered medical practitioner, who must have seen the patient within the past 24 hours.
Duration: up to *72 hours*.
Right of Appeal: none.
   Section 4 is rarely used in practice; it is potentially open to abuse and the Code of Practice advises that it should only be applied when Section 2 would involve unreasonable delay. Section 4 can be converted into Section 2 by adding another doctor's recommendation.

PATIENTS ALREADY IN HOSPITAL

Both Sections 2 and 3 can be applied to patients already in hospital. In emergencies, it is possible to use Section 5:

Section 5(2): Application in Respect of a Patient already in Hospital: a voluntary patient can be detained on the recommendation of one doctor, normally the responsible consultant or named deputy, for up to 72 hours.

Section 5(4): *Nurses' Holding Power*: a voluntary patient can be detained by a registered mental nurse for up to six hours until a doctor is found.

Section 5 may be converted into Section 2 or Section 3 by the appropriate medical and social work opinions.

PATIENTS IN THE COMMUNITY

Section 17: gives a detained patient leave of absence from hospital, either for a predetermined period or an open-ended trial of suitability for discharge. The responsible medical officer can impose any conditions considered necessary in the interests of the patient or for the protection of others, for example administration of depot injections by the community nurse. Patients can be recalled to hospital for health reasons, but the power of recall lapses if not used within six months.

Guardianship: a lesser known and possibly underused section of the Act allows a patient over 16 years old who is suffering from mental disorder to be placed under the supervision of a guardian, either a named individual or the local social services authority. Recommendation is made by two doctors, one approved, and the application by the nearest relative or an approved social worker. The order lasts six months and may be renewed for a further six months in the first instance and subsequently for one year at a time.

A Guardian may, for example, require the patient to reside at a specified place (not a hospital); require access to the patient to be given, at the patient's residence, to any doctor, approved social worker or other specified person; or require the patient to attend at specified places and times for medical treatment, occupation, education and training (but cannot compel the patient to accept the treatment offered).

A "Supervised Discharge Order"?

Following a number of recent instances of violent crimes committed by psychotic patients who have declined treatment, various proposals for increasing the powers of compulsory supervision and treatment for patients in the community are currently under discussion between the Royal College of Psychiatrists and the Department of Health. The Mental Health (Patients in the Community) Act is due to come into force in 1996. This is designed to ensure that patients who have been detained in hospital, and present a serious risk to themselves or others, receive appropriate after-care following discharge. A risk assessment, a care plan, a key worker, and clear review arrangements are required.

RELATIVES

The Act defines the nearest relative from a set list, beginning with spouse, child, parent and sibling in that order. Elder relatives take precedence in each category, as do relatives who live with or care for the patient. Cohabitees can be designated nearest relatives in some circumstances.

The nearest relative has the power to discharge a patient from Section 2. Section 3 cannot be applied if the nearest relative objects, but an objection can be overruled by a county court if considered unreasonable.

A relative is not legally permitted to consent to treatment on behalf of an adult patient, so consent from the nearest relative does not remove the necessity to apply the Act.

APPROVED SOCIAL WORKERS (ASWs)

These have been approved, following specific training, as competent in dealing with mental disorder. Only ASWs (not other social workers) can make application under the Act, and local authorities have a statutory obligation to provide an ASW service. ASWs have a responsibility to ensure that hospital admission is the most appropriate way of dealing with the case. When the nearest relative rather than an ASW makes the application for admission, the hospital managers must request a social work report as soon as possible.

POLICE POWERS

Section 136: allows a police constable who finds a person who appears to suffer from mental disorder in a place to which the public has access to remove him/her to a place of safety for assessment by an ASW, who would usually request medical examination by a police surgeon and a psychiatrist. The person must appear in immediate need of care and control, and detention must appear necessary in the person's own interests or for the protection of others. Although Section 136 lasts up to 72 hours, good practice requires it to be cancelled after the professional assessment and, if necessary, replaced by Section 2 or 3.

Section 135 allows a constable, on a Magistrate's Warrant, to enter premises to remove a patient to a place of safety for up to 72 hours, if there is reasonable cause to suspect that a person suffering from mental disorder is being ill-treated, neglected or not under proper control, or is unable to care for himself/herself and is living alone. It is used infrequently, as the constable in such a situation traditionally "smells gas" and effects an entry under common law.

MENTALLY ABNORMAL OFFENDERS

Several Sections of the Act deal with mentally disordered offenders (Ch 21). These Sections are mainly applied after consultation with colleagues such as a forensic psychiatrist and/or a probation officer. Compulsory psychiatric treatment under the Act cannot be given in the prison setting, but only after transfer to a psychiatric hospital.

Accused Persons

Section 35 remands an accused person awaiting trial or sentence to a specified hospital for *observation*, on evidence from one doctor of reason to suspect mental disorder; in practice it is mainly used for the preparation of psychiatric reports.

Section 36 remands a person accused of an imprisonable offence to hospital for *treatment*, on the evidence of two doctors, one of whom will be in charge of treatment. The patient must have a mental illness or severe mental impairment.

Both Sections 35 and 36 last *28 days*, renewable at 28-day intervals up to *12 weeks*.

Sentenced Persons

Section 37 permits a court to order hospital admission (or occasionally guardianship) for a patient, found guilty of an imprisonable offence except murder, who is suffering from mental disorder of a nature or degree which makes this course appropriate. Two doctors, one approved, must give evidence. It lasts up to *six months*, and may be renewed, appeal to a Mental Health Review Tribunal being allowed in the second six months.

Section 38: interim hospital order: allows a trial of psychiatric treatment for *three months* when a full Section 37 may be inappropriate.

A restriction order (*Section 41*) is infrequently applied in addition to Section 37, for serious cases in which the patient may not be given leave, transferred or discharged without permission from the Home Secretary (in practice, a particular branch of the Home Office) in order to protect the public. The Home Secretary may sometimes come under pressure from MPs or members of the public in relation to individual patients on restriction orders.

Section 47: transfer of a sentenced prisoner, and *Section 48: transfer of other prisoners* (*including remanded*) *to hospital*, by order of the Home Secretary, on two medical recommendations. A restriction on discharge may be added (*Section 49*) and applies until the end of the sentence with remission. The patient may appeal to a tribunal in the first six months.

CONSENT TO TREATMENT

Somewhat paradoxically, many detained patients consent to have treatment once they are "sectioned", but others do not.

Section 58: treatment requiring consent or a second opinion covers the use of ECT in detained patients, and administration of drugs when a particular medication is being continued longer than three months. Administration of such treatment requires that either:

- The patient consented and this has been certified as "informed" either by the responsible medical officer or an independent doctor,

or

- An independent doctor has certified that the patient has not given consent or is not capable of understanding the nature, purpose and likely effects of the treatment, but that having regard to the likelihood of its alleviating or preventing deterioration of his/her condition the treatment should be given. The independent doctor must consult two other staff members, one a nurse, the other neither a doctor nor a nurse.

Section 57: *treatment requiring consent* and *a second opinion*, covers the special conditions regulating two treatments which have often given rise to ethical concern: *psychosurgery*, and *surgical implantation of hormones to reduce male sexual drive*.

Here, the patient's informed consent is not sufficient on its own (whether the patient is detained or voluntary). It must be supported by an independent doctor appointed by the Mental Health Act Commission, and two other non-medical appointed persons who have certified in writing that the patient is capable of understanding the nature, purpose and likely effects of the proposed treatment and has consented to it. This occasionally gives rise to situations where a patient consents to, or even requests, a particular treatment (for example hormone treatment of a sex offender) but the Commission refuses.

Section 62: *urgent treatment*: a treatment normally restricted under Sections 57 or 58 may be given to a detained patient without obtaining formal consent or a second opinion in an emergency, for example ECT to save the life of a seriously dehydrated depressed patient. In practice, such treatment would often be given under common law.

INFORMATION FOR DETAINED PATIENTS

Section 132 specifies the duties of hospital managers to inform detained patients as soon as possible, both orally and in writing, about their legal position and their rights of appeal.

Detained Patients' Rights of Appeal

There is an initial right of appeal to the *hospital managers*: unless there has been procedural irregularity, it is unusual for managers to over-rule clinicians.

Subsequent appeal is to a *Mental Health Review Tribunal*, which consists of three members: a lawyer (the chairperson), a doctor and a lay person. Tribunals may discharge detained patients if they consider them no longer dangerous or no longer suffering from mental disorder. They may also recommend leave of absence, or transfer to another hospital. Patients under certain Sections have the right of application to a tribunal. Review by a tribunal is mandatory at specified intervals for some of the longer treatment Sections, such as Section 3, and must be requested by the hospital managers if the patient has not already exercised the right to a tribunal hearing.

Patients may be eligible for Legal Aid to assist them in preparing a case, to obtain an independent medical opinion and to cover the cost of legal representation.

MENTAL HEALTH ACT COMMISSION

This is a special Health Authority multidisciplinary body, its members including doctors, nurses, social workers, lawyers and lay persons. Its function is to see that detained patients are being cared for appropriately and that the Mental Health Act is being properly applied. Members visit every psychiatric unit in the country once or twice a year, and every Special Hospital at least once a month, to see detained patients, ensure the staff are adhering to the principles of the Act, and consider any complaints which have arisen. Appointed members provide independent second opinions.

FURTHER READING

Bluglass R (1983) *A Guide to the Mental Health Act*. Churchill Livingstone: Edinburgh
Department of Health and Welsh Office (1990) *Code of Practice: Section 118 of the Mental Health Act 1983*. HMSO: London
Jones R (ed) (1994) *Mental Health Act Manual* (4th edn). Sweet & Maxwell: London

Glossary of Terms

This Glossary defines some technical terms used to describe phenomena of mental illness and concepts of psychotherapy.

Abreaction: The recall to consciousness of a repressed trauma, with a re-experiencing of the emotion which originally accompanied it. Achievement of abreaction (catharsis) may be through psychotherapy alone, hypnosis, or drugs, usually barbiturates or amphetamines.

Acting out: Repetition of a maladaptive behaviour pattern as a substitute for verbal acknowledgement of the underlying emotions during psychotherapy.

Affect: Mood.

Agitation: Motor restlessness, usually accompanied by subjective anxiety. Occurs in anxiety states and depressive illness.

Akathisia: Motor restlessness due to malfunction of the extrapyramidal system. A side-effect of antipsychotic drugs.

Alexithymia: Inability to verbalise emotions. Postulated as a predisposing factor for somatisation disorders.

Amnesia: Loss of memory. May be due to organic brain disease, e.g. Alzheimer's disease, Korsakov's syndrome; or to functional psychiatric conditions, e.g. dissociative disorder, depressive illness.

Asthenic: Weak, inadequate.

Asyndetic thinking: Absence of logical connection between topics. May occur in schizophrenia. Synonymous with knight's move thinking.

Autism: (1) Autistic thinking: the subject is absorbed in personal fantasies or delusions, and his or her thoughts are divorced from external reality. May occur in schizophrenia.
(2) Childhood autism: a form of childhood psychosis.

Autochthonous delusion: see Delusion.

Borderline: (1) A term used by psychotherapists to describe patients on the brink of psychosis.
(2) A personality type included in DSM-IV.

Catatonia: Mutism and immobility without impairment of consciousness. Occurs in schizophrenia.

Catharsis: Achievement of abreaction.

Circumstantiality: Excessively detailed and lengthy thought or talk which wanders round the point. Sometimes associated with epilepsy, low intelligence or obsessional personality.

Compulsion: An obsessional act, which subject carries out despite trying to resist doing so.

Confabulation: Elaborate falsifications, probably believed by the subject, which cover up defects of memory. Occurs in amnesic states especially Korsakov's syndrome.

Conversion: The manifestation of repressed emotion in the form of bodily symptoms (conversion hysteria).

Countertransference: See Transference.

Cyclothymic: A personality type prone to variation in mood.

Delirium: Acute clouding of consciousness often accompanied by delusions and hallucinations, due to organic brain disease.

Delusion: An incorrigible false belief, inconsistent with the information available and with the beliefs of the subject's social group. Delusions may occur in the functional psychoses and some organic states. Paranoid delusions are the most common type. Delusions in accord with the prevailing affect may occur in the affective disorders, e.g. delusions of guilt, nihilistic, or hypochondriacal delusions in depression, and grandiose delusions in mania. Other types are religious and sexual delusions.
　　Primary (autochthonous) delusions suddenly enter consciousness fully formed, sometimes preceded by a period of "delusional

mood", and are among the first rank symptoms of schizophrenia. They may take the form of a delusional perception, developing in conjunction with an ordinary sense perception; a delusional memory; or a delusional awareness. Secondary delusions are often elaborated from them.

Dementia: Chronic, usually irreversible, impairment of cognitive function due to organic brain disease.

Denial: Inability to accept unpalatable material, including self-knowledge and/or external events. An unconscious means of avoiding distress.

Depersonalisation: A sensation of dream-like unreality of the self. Usually secondary to an anxiety state or depressive illness, but may occur on its own in young people.

Depression: (1) A mood state characterised by sadness, not necessarily pathological.
(2) Depressive illness.

Derealisation: A sensation of dream-like unreality of the outside world. Occurs in association with depersonalisation.

Displacement: The transfer of emotion from the person or object which caused it towards a different but more acceptable one.

Dissociation: A splitting of consciousness in which some part of mental function becomes disconnected from the rest, e.g. amnesia for a distressing event.

Dysmorphophobia: An exaggerated belief that part of the body looks abnormal.

Echolalia and Echopraxia: The subject imitates the speech and actions of others.

Ego: The part of the self, largely conscious, which deals with reality.

Elation: Elevation of mood, either in normal people or secondary to mental illness, e.g. mania or schizophrenia.

Euphoria: An exaggerated sense of well-being, usually indicating organic cerebral dysfunction.

Fixation: Arrest of one or more aspects of personality development at a stage of incomplete maturity.

Flight of ideas: Sudden changes in train of thought arising from incidental connections between words or ideas, like rhymes or puns. Occurs in mania.

Fugue: A state of altered consciousness in which the subject wanders away. May occur in depressive illness, dissociative disorders, post-epileptic states, drug- or alcohol-induced states, and after head injury.

Functional: A term applied to psychiatric disorders for which no biological cause has been found and which are presumed to be due to psychological factors.

Hallucination: A false perception arising in the absence of an appropriate external stimulus. Hallucinations occur in both "functional psychoses" and organic brain syndromes. Auditory, visual, tactile, somatic, olfactory and gustatory types exist. Auditory ones in the form of voices are most frequent. Specific types of third person voices are characteristic of schizophrenia. Second person voices occur in many disorders, but in the affective disorders the content tends to accord with the patient's mood.

Hypochondriasis: Excessive concern about health.

Id: A primitive, largely unconscious part of the self, motivated by instinct and seeking gratification.

Ideas of reference: Misinterpretation of external events as referring to the subject, usually in a derogatory way. Occur in paranoid states, but also in self-conscious young people without psychiatric illness.

Identification: Conscious or unconscious assumption of the characteristics of another person, usually someone admired by the subject.

Illusion: A perceptual distortion whereby a stimulus is misinterpreted. May occur in normal people or be secondary to mental illness.

Incongruity of affect: The subject's emotions are inappropriate to the circumstances. Characteristic of schizophrenia, but may occur in affective disorders or organic states.

Introjection: The process by which the characteristics of another person, or "external object", are incorporated by the subject in the process of personality development.

Knight's move thinking: See Asyndetic thinking.

Libido: (1) Sexual drive.
(2) General psychic energy.

Mannerisms: Artificial or exaggerated modes of speech or movement.

Negativism: Carrying out actions of an opposite nature to those that are requested or seem appropriate.

Neologism: An idiosyncratic word which has a personal meaning for the subject. May occur in schizophrenia.

Neuroses: A group of psychiatric illnesses in which delusions and hallucinations do not occur and the symptoms often represent an exaggeration of normal response to stress. Insight and contact with reality are usually retained. Synonymous with "psycho-neuroses".

Obsession: A recurrent idea or impulse which enters consciousness despite resistance by the subject.

Oedipal: Concerned with an unconscious desire for the parent of opposite sex, combined with hostility towards the same-sex parent. Applied to children of both sexes, though strictly speaking "Oedipus complex" should be used for boys and "Electra complex" for girls.

Overinclusive thinking: The subject's sense of concept boundaries is blurred, so ideas with little relevance to the topic are included, and thought becomes vague. May occur in schizophrenia.

Overvalued idea: An idea held with great conviction, but differing from a delusion in that it is not necessarily false, and the subject is to some extent prepared to modify it in accordance with evidence. Associated with paranoid personality disorder.

Paranoid states: Conditions in which delusions or overvalued ideas, usually of persecutory content, are prominent.

Parapraxes: Slips of the tongue, lapses of memory or other minor mistakes, which seem to reveal unconscious feelings.

Passivity phenomena: Control of the subject's thoughts, emotions, or bodily actions is attributed to an outside agency. Characteristic of schizophrenia.

Perseveration: Continued repetition of speech or activity. Occurs in organic brain syndromes.

Phobia: An excessive fear of a particular object or situation.

Pressure of speech: Rapid speech, secondary to rapid thought of excess content. Occurs in mania.

Projection: Displacement of personal shortcomings or unacceptable emotions onto other people or outside factors. An unconscious means of avoiding guilt.

Pseudodementia: Impaired cognitive function secondary to a reversible functional illness such as depression.

Pseudohallucination: A false perception, visual or auditory, which appears to be located in the subject's "inner space" rather than to be coming from the external world, and is recognised as unreal by the subject.

Psychoses: A group of psychiatric conditions in which the symptoms, e.g. delusions and hallucinations, are qualitatively different from normal experiences. There is often loss of insight, loss of contact with reality, and deterioration of the personality. "Organic" psychoses result from physical factors affecting the brain, whereas in "functional" psychoses the cause is unknown.

Psychosomatic: Physiological dysfunction secondary to mental factors.

Rationalisation: The subject explains his actions by a logical or admirable motive when the true one is less edifying.

Reaction formation: An unacceptable feeling is repressed, and the subject gives expression to its opposite.

Regression: A reversion to thoughts, feelings, or behaviour appropriate to an earlier stage of maturation.

Repression: Unacceptable thoughts or impulses are excluded from conscious awareness.

Resistance: Opposition to interpretations of unconscious material during psychotherapy.

Retardation: (1) Psychomotor retardation: slowing of speech and motor activity.
(2) Mental retardation: an older term for learning disability.

Somatisation: Expression of emotional distress in the guise of physical complaints.

Stereotypy: A meaningless, bizarre repetitive action. May occur in schizophrenia.

Sublimation: The redirection of frustrated desires into socially acceptable channels.

Superego: The self-critical part of the self, developed through introjection of parental standards.

Thought block: Sudden interruption of the train of thought. Occurs in schizophrenia.

Thought interference: The subject's own thoughts are believed to be inserted, withdrawn, or broadcast by some external agency. Characteristic of schizophrenia.

Transference: Emotions which the subject experienced towards someone in the past are projected onto another person. Often used in the context of a patient's feelings towards a psychotherapist. "Countertransference" is the equivalent in reverse, the therapist's feelings for the patient.

Verbigeration: Constant repetition of a single word or phrase. May occur in schizophrenia.

Word salad: A mixture of neologisms which renders speech incomprehensible. May occur in schizophrenia.

FURTHER READING

Kraupl Taylor F (1983) Descriptive and Developmental Phenomena. In *Handbook of Psychiatry 1: General Psychopathology* (eds M Shepherd, OL Zangwill). Cambridge University Press: Cambridge

Walton H (ed) *Dictionary of Psychiatry*. Blackwell Scientific Publications: Oxford

Index

Note: **Bold** numbers indicate major references.

Index compiled by Susan Ramsey